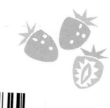

Contents

Advance Praise for *Superfruits*

"Paul Gross's straightforward and well-documented book provides strong direction and clear-cut answers for consumers, based on well-reasoned research and compelling evidence. His use of . . . superfruits criteria and a 'points system' for rating health-beneficial fruits is a welcome answer to consumers seeking the best choices for themselves and their families."

—Mary Ann Lila Ph.D., director, Plants for Human Health Institute, North Carolina State University

"Paul Gross, the 'Berry Doctor,' goes beyond the marketing hype on superfruits, using an easy-to-understand method of ranking potential stars. By looking at nutrient density, research support, and popular appeal, Gross delivers a cornucopia of offerings that can easily enhance well-being . . . whether via simple suggestions in the breakdown of each offering, a list of the types of products to look for in the supermarket, or by following the creative recipes from the back of the book."

—Heather Granato, group editor, Virgo Publishing

"This is a book for the public, for nutritionists, M.D.s, alternative medical practitioners, vegetarians—for anyone who wants to better understand what a well-chosen selection of superfruits can do for you inside and out besides tasting great."

—Ian Crown, Panoramic Fruit Company, Puerto Rico

"Dr. Gross is a leading expert and strong proponent of consumer education and superfruit science, and following careers as a university scientist, entrepreneur, and food industry consultant, he is the leading advocate for superfruits and superfruit science."

—Steve Talcott Ph.D., Department of Food Chemistry, Texas A&M University

Superfruits

PAUL GROSS, Ph.D.
THE "BERRY DOCTOR"

New York Chicago San Francisco Lisbon London Madrid Mexico City
Milan New Delhi San Juan Seoul Singapore Sydney Toronto

Library of Congress Cataloging-in-Publication Data

Gross, Paul M.
    Superfruits / by Paul Gross.
        p.   cm.
    Includes bibliographical references and index.
    ISBN 13: 978-0-07-163387-1 (alk. paper)
    ISBN 10: 0-07-163387-1 (alk. paper)
    1. Fruit in human nutrition.   2. Fruit.   3. Smoothies (Beverages)   I. Title.

QP144.F78G76   2010
613.2—dc22   2009017479

For family—Lil, Cam, Phil, Frank—*each an inspiration*

1 2 3 4 5 6 7 8 9 10 11 12 13 14 15 16 17 18 19 20 21 22 23 24   DOC/DOC   0 9

ISBN   978-0-07-163387-1
MHID   0-07-163387-1

Interior design by Monica Baziuk

McGraw-Hill books are available at special quantity discounts to use as premiums and sales promotions or for use in corporate training programs. To contact a representative, please e-mail us at bulksales@mcgraw-hill.com.

The information contained in this book is intended to provide helpful and informative material on the subject addressed. It is not intended to serve as a replacement for professional medical advice. Any use of the information in this book is at the reader's discretion. The author and publisher disclaim any and all liability arising directly or indirectly from the use or application of any information contained in this book.

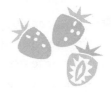

Foreword

I CONSIDER IT A great privilege to work in the world of fruits and, each day, conduct research trials on fruits harvested from locations both near and far. When I think of people eating fruit, I have a mental image of warm, happy days, smiles on faces, and looks of pure enjoyment. I experience this sense of pleasure daily with my own family in our frequent trips to the community fruit bowl or our well-stocked refrigerator filled with seasonal and nonseasonal fruits and juices. A quick look around your local supermarket will readily reveal that the fruits and juices of our childhood memories have changed. We now have new, improved, and exotic products to choose from, many claiming to be "super" good for you. The choices can be overwhelming—and, after all, what does an açaí berry, goji berry, or blackcurrant taste like, and should I spend my hard-earned money to buy it?

This all leads to a valid and thought-provoking question: Are all fruits created equal, or are some fruits created "super"? If there are indeed "superfruits," can we apply logic and infer that there are also "not-so-super" fruits?

As a food chemist, I conduct research on phytochemical compounds in fruits responsible for their color, flavor, and potential health benefits. I know that all fruits inherently contain some level of nutrients, that not all varieties of the same fruits are the same, and that all contain at least some nonnutrient compounds known as phytochemicals that may contribute directly or indirectly to our overall health and wellness. To use a simple analogy: as someone who works with many different fruits, deciding between super or not-super fruits is like asking a mother to choose a favorite from among her children. So, when it comes to fruits, we need to realize that each one has something unique to offer our palates and our bodies. Those unique properties may be energy, a preferred taste or aroma, dietary fiber, hunger, satiety, or what we hope will be a positive benefit on our overall health.

What, then, is a "superfruit," and why do we see so many fruits that seemingly compete for the right to be called "super"? The reality is that most scientists do not use the term *superfruit* or *superfood*, but rather these terms came to international prominence via a route that bypassed the research laboratory or government regulatory agency. There is nothing inherently wrong with the term *superfruit*; as consumers, we are often persuaded to purchase products based on a well-conceived marketing program. Simply put, from time to time, nature gives us fruits in abundance that science can define as superior to others in delivering both nutrient and nonnutrient compounds.

A browse through your local supermarket or specialty foods store over the past years has no doubt been an adventurous endeavor. Unless you reside in a major metropolitan area or spend extensive time traveling abroad, your earlier experience with fruits such as pomegranate, mango, açaí, goji berry, mangosteen, and papaya was likely quite limited, yet in today's superfruit world you can enjoy these fruits routinely, and often in various formats—fresh, juiced, dried, or blended into beverages. The marketing messages from these fruits can also be overwhelming and may be based on an exaggeration of the limited research studies conducted on the actual fruit. As an upshot, consumers are now accustomed to mention of such obscure substances as antioxidants, polyphenolics, carotenoids, anthocyanins, omega-3 fatty acids, and resveratrol, which are used as buzzwords to gain market attention and hold consumer interest.

As a fruit scientist, I readily admit that we know far too little about the direct health benefits of fruit consumption, not to mention those fruits categorized as superfruits, but fortunately for us all, Dr. Paul Gross has taken on the daunting challenge to reveal the elusive world of superfruits in this entertaining and informative book. Dr. Gross is a leading expert and strong proponent of consumer education and superfruit science, and following careers as a university scientist, entrepreneur, and food industry consultant, he is the leading advocate for superfruits and superfruit science. Affectionately referred to as "the Berry Doctor," Dr. Gross has educated countless people, including scientists and medical professionals, on the richness and benefits that superfruits bring to our lives.

In this book, Dr. Gross will take you through a set of five simple criteria that he uses to create a ranked list of twenty fruits to which he refers as nature's top superfruits. He freely admits that no one fruit will provide all of the nutrients that our bodies need, yet he shows us that consuming whole foods (and lots of them) can be one of the most important contributing aspects of a healthy lifestyle. His inclusion criteria were wisely established based on factors such as nutrient and nonnutrient content, biomedical research, and the ability to eventually file for government-approved health claims, as well as critical subjective qualities, such as packaging, flavor, affordability, and availability to the consumer.

The last point I want to make regarding fruits, vegetables, and even superfruits is that the only way to gain their benefits is to actually consume them. Trends from around the world show few positive changes in the overall health status of populations and indicate that our diets are still lacking in sufficient intake of fruits, vegetables, and whole grains. I concede that there is no simple solution to our dietary inadequacies and that consuming superfruits may be an answer to this dilemma. Perhaps the "Age of the Superfruit" is now upon us, and superfruits have the ability to offer novelty, diversity, and intrigue to encourage healthier lifestyles and dietary habits.

STEVE TALCOTT, PH.D.
Associate Professor of Food Chemistry
Texas A&M University

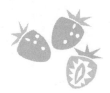

Acknowledgments

CONCEPTS FOR THIS BOOK came from my experiences as a youth in Chatham, Ontario, Canada, overlapped with American and British university education, research training, and professional development as a health scientist. Life lessons from all three countries led to my interest in nutrition, phytochemicals, and how "super" fruits can offer a solution for healthier dietary practices.

Special thanks to Fiona Sarne of McGraw-Hill, for her vision of the book's place in the public, streamlined editing, and efficient organization of resources; Ian Crown of Stamford, Connecticut, and Panoramic Fruit Company, Puerto Rico, for years of good humor and entertaining education through the eyes of a fruit horticulturalist; and Steve Talcott, Ph.D., of Texas A&M University, for challenging my ideas, critiquing early drafts, and providing active research leadership in superfruit science.

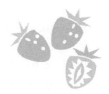

Introduction
Welcome to the World of Superfruits!

I N THE PAST FEW years, the word *superfruit* has blared into the headlines with alluring fanfare. What began as just a few curious exotic juices in the American market has now evolved into thousands of products in a multibillion-dollar global industry. From the start, the superfruit category has been more about marketing than science. Beverages made from rare, enchanting fruit species marketed with a message of antioxidant benefits have beckoned consumers with a seductive array of irresistible health promises.

The truth is that some fruits proposed as "super" really aren't, and no claims about antioxidant health benefits from fruits are actually established by science or allowed by regulatory authorities. I'm going to expose some misconceptions about this expanding category of superfoods and give you a list of twenty fruits that are *actually super* based on nutritional facts and scientific criteria. I'll share with you how these twenty superfruits can be easily added to your diet, not just because they are delicious, but also for their nutrient properties—scientifically proved to have the potential for lowering your risk of contracting major diseases.

This book stems from my teaching and research career in physiology—the branch of biological sciences specializing in how organs of the body work together moment by moment throughout life. This pursuit demands an understanding of how foods are digested to supply essential nutrients, which are then circulated via the blood to nourish all of the body's organs and cells. Nutrient-rich whole superfruits can give your body a headstart for making this process efficient and easy to repeat through practice of a healthy diet over all years of your life.

As a physiologist, I am also interested in why organs fail and disease develops. Having been a research director in a university hospital surgery department and cofounder of a clinical trials management company, I have been close enough to major diseases to know that many are preventable by healthy living practices, including the right nutritional content and amount of food. In nearly every developed country today, however, there is a spiraling trend of obesity and its constellation of associated diseases such as chronic inflammation and pain, diabetes, blood and cardiovascular disorders, psychological illnesses, and even several types of cancer—many of these related to poor nutritional content and excessive food intake.

This book will show you how to use superfruits as delicious, *whole-food* sources of essential nutrients your body requires for general well-being.

The Truth About Superfruit Juices

By my definition, superfruits should be all about sustaining regular healthy intake of *nutrients from whole foods*, not processed, blended, and diluted juices—a definition that may be surprising to you. Did you know that most of the juices that stimulated the concept of superfruits are highly processed so that there is little left in them except color and taste? They are marketed on myths of ancient uses for unproved health benefits, not on the nutrient value of the natural fruit that this book emphasizes.

You may have come to this book looking for insights about exotic fruits renowned as top antioxidant superfruit juices. This subject will be addressed but perhaps with unexpected truths. The base of science for most existing superfruit products has not been adequately explained, leaving a knowledge gap between actual fruit compounds in the product and the health value expected from them. We're going to get the facts about superfruits straight in this book!

My message is that superfruits should be your constant reminder and daily source of *nutrients*. Contrary to the way superfruits are marketed currently—as antioxidant-rich juices—this book is about *whole* fruits truly superior due to their natural high density of scientifically established nutrients essential for maintaining health.

What About Pills or Supplements as Substitutes for Superfruits?

There will always be someone looking for a simpler solution. I've heard it many times: "Why not devise a pill or just a scoop of powder that contains all those nutrients and interesting phytochemicals from a few of your favorite superfruits? Wouldn't that be a popular product in the diet world?"

In the industry of nutraceuticals—extracts from natural sources thought to have a beneficial effect—quite a few manufacturers actually take on this challenge and make a supplement of green or purple powder that supposedly simplifies food intake into a single serving. As a proponent of a whole-food diet, I have a few thoughts about such products that challenge this logic:

► How do you know that the proportions of nutrients and phytochemicals in the whole natural superfruit are preserved?
► The phytochemical "synergy," as discussed in Part I, is compromised by processing a whole fruit into a pill or powder. The manufacturer makes the choice about which nutrients to include. Can it be better than nature has done in whole superfruits? I say no.
► One of the superfruit signature nutrients with broad health effects—prebiotic dietary fiber (also called soluble or viscous fiber)—is manufactured *out* of nearly every pill or capsule, unless purposely put back in. Don't miss out on the important health values of prebiotic fiber.
► Superfruits not only are highly nutritious and enjoyable to eat but also furnish calories for your energy needs during the day. Giving that up for the convenience of a pill or supplement defeats a purpose for consuming whole foods—obtaining calories for our day's physical activity needs.
► There are undeniable pleasures in eating whole foods—their fragrance, taste, juiciness, crunch, and feeling of freshness—that pills and powders can never match.
► Cost: why deny all of the foregoing benefits for a pill or powder at a price usually higher than the natural whole superfruit?

How Do Fruits Earn "Super" Status?

So, what is it that sets superfruits apart from regular fruits or currently marketed superfruit juices? I believe it's an optimal mix of natural fruit compounds—nutrients and phytochemicals—that should be in everyone's diet.

My choices of top superfruits come by looking in each fruit for natural nutrient groups: (1) the antioxidant vitamins A (from plant compounds called carotenoids), C, and E; (2) B vitamins; (3) essential dietary minerals; (4) amino acids and protein; (5) dietary fiber, both soluble and insoluble; (6) omega fats; and (7) phytosterols. These are natural nutrients for growth of the fruit itself—how it was designed in nature throughout evolution—that are known from modern physiological studies on diets to be essential to human health. Any whole fruit containing them all in rich amounts would indeed be super!

Also included among my valued superfruit characteristics are two classes of nonnutrient phytochemicals called carotenoids and polyphenols (also known as phenolics or phenolic acids). Both classes include natural color chemicals called pigments, consisting of hundreds to thousands of individual compounds giving color and other qualities to plants. Carotenoids and polyphenols are under intensive research for their potential health values to humans.

Many advocates of superfruit juices believe they are getting a whole-fruit serving (or more, in some exaggerated cases!) by consuming one serving of juice. It's not always the case. Let's look at the accompanying table to see how processing from a whole fruit (edible portions such as pulp, skin, and seeds) to its juice diminishes nutrient and phytochemical levels.

Clear from this table is that juice processing can steal away nutrients and food value of natural whole fruits. Often such juices also must be sweetened with excessive sugar or other common fruit juices to offset their natural acidity and sourness. Flavor may benefit from these procedures, but nutrient content suffers. Especially detrimental is that juice processing eliminates the digestive health value of the fruit's natural fiber content—the two kinds of dietary fiber providing many valuable health benefits for you.

WHAT'S MISSING FROM SUPERFRUIT JUICES THAT WHOLE FRUITS NATURALLY CONTAIN?

Nutrients	Content in Whole Superfruits	Content in Superfruit Juices	Comments on Content
Vitamins A-C-E	high	low or absent	vulnerable and diminished by processing
B vitamins	high	low or absent	vulnerable and diminished by processing
Essential minerals	high	low or unknown	variably affected by processing
Amino acids and protein	moderate–high	low or absent	vulnerable and diminished by processing
Prebiotic (soluble) fiber	moderate–high	low or absent	vulnerable and diminished by processing
Insoluble fiber	high	absent	eliminated
Omega fatty acids	depends on fruit source	absent	eliminated
Phytosterols	depends on fruit source	low or absent	vulnerable and diminished by processing
Edible seeds	depends on fruit source	absent	eliminated
Edible skin	depends on fruit source	absent	eliminated
Polyphenols	depends on fruit source	diminished	vulnerable to processing
Carotenoids	depends on fruit source	diminished	vulnerable to processing

Notwithstanding, some superfruit juices are fine to include in your diet—ones that are clearly labeled "100 percent pure juice," having no (or minimal) other ingredients. Although I'm a proponent of eating the fresh fruit itself, some juices are still a good way to get *partial* nutrients that superfruits offer. In later sections of the book, I suggest specific superfruit juice products that aren't completely diminished of the potential health benefits that whole fruits offer.

Twenty *True* Superfruits

It's time to introduce you to nature's top twenty whole fruits that are truly "super." From what criteria did I create this list? These were factors that first caught my interest in superfruits, but I wanted to apply objective criteria for defining true superfruits. More details will be given in Part II. For now, criteria for superfruit status can be summarized by five factors:

► Nutrient diversity and density
► Phytochemical diversity and density
► Basic research intensity
► Clinical research progress
► Popularity based on sensory appeal and market demand

So, let's see the list of nature's top twenty superfruits. I'll be explaining each one in Part II, where I give a points system based on the preceding five criteria to assign a superfruit score and rank.

1. Mango
2. Fig
3. Orange
4. Strawberry
5. Goji (wolfberry)
6. Red grape
7. Cranberry
8. Kiwifruit
9. Papaya
10. Blueberry
11. Cherry, sweet and tart species
12. Red raspberry
13. Seaberry (seabuckthorn)
14. Guava
15. Blackberry
16. Blackcurrant
17. Date
18. Pomegranate
19. Açaí
20. Dried plum (prune)

Superfruits and Health Research

You may have encountered the word *superfruit* in various places in the media, but scientists don't apply the word in any research report. This is a marketing term used by manufacturers to attract attention to their products, but it's been accepted by the fruit processing industry and by consumers, so it has become a convenient way to refer to fruits with special qualities. I want to emphasize *whole food* superfruits as important to have regularly in your diet, hopefully to make a positive difference to your current health and lower your risk of diseases. This means we have to pay attention to how research is identifying health criteria and benefits from eating superfruits.

By tracking the research literature on fruits over the past few years, I was able to see progress in the scientific understanding regarding each of the top twenty superfruits. While each has been given coverage in industry reports and the general consumer media, the amount of background medical research on these fruits has varied from fruit to fruit, but overall it is astounding. Some two thousand reports on the twenty superfruits have been published in scientific journals in *each* year since the middle of this decade! That's more than eight thousand research projects on superfruits just since the category was first mentioned in 2004.

Of more interest is the substantial growing investment in clinical trials (human studies specifically testing antidisease effects) on some superfruits. Early in 2009, ninety active clinical studies on fruits from the preceding list were registered in the United States and around the world.

A Health Claims Research Pyramid

Like Indiana Jones, virtually every manufacturer of a superfruit product is hot on the trail of the Holy Grail—a health claim approved by a national regulatory agency such as the U.S. Food and Drug Administration (FDA) or European Food Safety Authority (EFSA). In simple terms, a health claim would verify that the product or compound has been scientifically proved to have a direct effect on health or the specific ability to alter the course of a disease.

How does a fruit or extract get to this lofty position in health research? All candidates for a health claim must pass through an arduous, long-duration series of four steps, as shown in the accompanying pyramid.

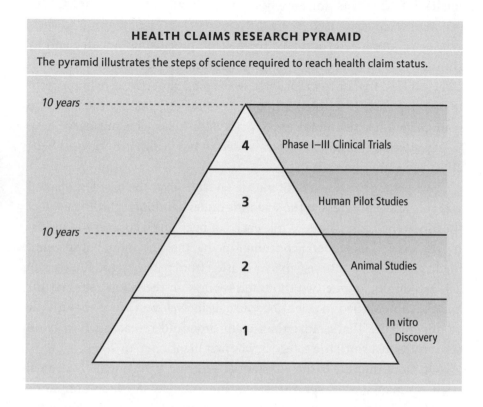

HEALTH CLAIMS RESEARCH PYRAMID

The pyramid illustrates the steps of science required to reach health claim status.

10 years

4 — Phase I–III Clinical Trials

3 — Human Pilot Studies

10 years

2 — Animal Studies

1 — In vitro Discovery

1. At the base of the pyramid are experiments in the laboratory using in vitro ("in glass") experiments to define initial properties of an agent with unknown properties. Tests are done on isolated cells or in vitro model systems, sometimes including a specific disease model, such as cultured cancer cells.
2. The next step in the pyramid comprises tests on animals to see the actions of the undefined compound in a living organism, also called in vivo ("in life"). Because the same procedures from the in vitro studies need to be replicated in vivo, nearly all animal experiments depend on previously established in vitro results. Called "basic research," steps 1 and 2 typically require ten years of integrated investigation and have a high degree of failure. The major-

ity of fruits (or their extracts) called superfruits in the media or in product promotions are actually still within the bottom half of the pyramid and so, by this criterion, have not yet accomplished sufficient research to be called *super*.

3. Ascending the pyramid, step 3 is the place for "first-in-human" pilot studies, in which an exploratory dose, a specific biomarker for a physiological response, or tracer studies will be examined. For most true superfruits in advanced research, this is the current level of progress.

4. The peak of the pyramid is where all the previous research gets focused on testing for a specific health effect in humans—usually subjects having a disease that the test agent may relieve. Success here would mean that the health claim can eventually specify that this fruit or extract "may reduce the risk of cancer" or another disease.

A complete step-4 program is achieved through three stages in human testing called phase I–III clinical trials, which specifically determine whether a health benefit (or antidisease action) occurs. This testing is often called "clinical research." The fastest a tested compound can go through a complete step 4 is about ten years.

Where are some superfruits and extracts that are under current medical research located within the research pyramid? In the abbreviated list of fruits and extracts that follows, you can readily see that some superfruits—açaí berries, blueberries, and strawberries—are still in basic research within the bottom half of the pyramid (ten-plus years from qualifying for human research requirements), whereas other superfruits—cranberries, red grapes, the grape extract resveratrol, and anthocyanins extracted from different fruits—are progressing through clinical research within step 4.

Potential Health Benefits of Superfruits

Just what are some of the potential benefits for maintaining health and lowering the risk of diseases provided by a whole-food diet involving superfruits? The complete picture has not been filled in yet, but active scientific research on the twenty superfruits shows progress for minimizing the risk of certain diseases, as shown in the accompanying list.

POSITION WITHIN THE RESEARCH PYRAMID

Fruit or extract	Step position in pyramid	Year for reaching step 4	Forecast year for earliest possible health claim approval
Açaí berries	1	2014	> 2020
Anthocyanins	3	2010	2014
Blueberries	2	2012	> 2020
Cranberries	4	2008	2012
Red grapes	4	2008	2012
Resveratrol	4	2008	2012
Strawberries	2	2014	> 2020

Forecasts are estimates based on current basic research and clinical trial activity.

The four at the top—cardiovascular disorders (heart disease, high blood pressure, vascular disease, stroke), inflammation and pain (such as chronic arthritis), several types of cancer, and antibacterial effects—are where superfruit research has made the most progress. For example, separate clinical studies with red grapes, cranberries, pomegranates, oranges, or any extract of these fruits are closest to achieving FDA- or EFSA-approved confirmation for specifically acting against a human disease. Here's the list of just some health problems that superfruits may deter:

► Cardiovascular diseases
► Inflammation and pain
► Several types of cancer
► Microbial, fungal, parasitic, and viral infections
► Metabolic syndrome, obesity, and diabetes
► Gastrointestinal and digestive disorders
► Symptoms of premature aging such as neurological disorders
► Immune deficiencies and allergies
► Osteoporosis
► Skin and dental disorders

Superfruits and the Color Code

Incorporating colorful plant foods in your diet can be simplified by picturing them in four color groups, as proposed in a dietary plan called the Color Code (see Appendix D for citations):

- ▶ Orange-yellow
- ▶ Red-tan
- ▶ Blue-purple-black
- ▶ Green

It's very similar to the advice of government health organizations encouraging us to eat "five-a-day" portions of fruits and vegetables having different colors. Superfruit colors fit conveniently into a Color Code plan, so I'll be using this format in Part III as a guide for shopping and meal planning with superfruits.

There's a good scientific basis for using the Color Code to remind yourself about whole-food superfruits. I mentioned the pigment phytochemicals called carotenoids and polyphenols (particularly including anthocyanins), which together provide colors of all plant foods that we easily recognize—such as oranges and lemons; red apples and strawberries; purple grapes and blueberries; and dark green mangoes, guavas, or spinach. These pigments are hotly pursued research subjects in hundreds of current studies in food science, biotechnology, and clinical research. Similar to shopping for superfruits by their colors, scientists are attracted to color-rich plant foods to analyze pigments that research shows may have promising health benefits.

However, interest for medical research is not the main purpose of the Color Code. Keeping it simple, the Color Code is for shopping and meal planning! Fruits with bright colors that appeal to the eye are at their peak ripeness and optimal production of compounds having nutritional value to you. Because superfruits are the most nutrient-rich of fruits, it is also easier to shop for them and plan your meals according to a Color Code. I'll teach you how in Part III.

Putting Superfruits in Your Shopping Cart

You might be like me when grocery shopping: the fresh produce area is my favorite part of the store. It's where I can see the variety of colors, fragrances, shapes, and species of nature's gifts of fruits. Really, when it comes to stimulating the senses, nothing beats the fruit section!

As just stated, this is what I call shopping by the Color Code for four main color groups: orange-yellow, red-tan, blue-purple-black, and green. For fruits, those colors include nearly everything and therefore can become your guide if you adopt one simple suggestion: shopping by the Color Code means putting at least three superfruits of *different colors* in your basket each time you visit the fresh produce section. It's that easy! I'll show you the best way to shop for the top twenty superfruits and give you tips about certain superfruit product formats and other suggestions for getting these fruits into your cart . . . and into your diet!

Including Superfruits in Your Daily Diet

When people hear about factual advances in health research, they often look for ways to personally gain those benefits as soon as a viable product is available. So, how can everyone benefit most from investment in research advances on fruits? Eat more of them!

The central message here is that eating whole plant foods such as nutrient-rich superfruits is clearly an important part of a good diet, but variety matters as much as quantity. The key to sustainable health and enjoyment from your diet lies in regularly using a variety of whole fruits, especially those that really are super because of their nutrient diversity and density, phytochemical content, and potential to improve health and lower disease risk. This way, you're not only maximizing the variety of nutrient values from different fruits but also leveraging the best information from research on how they can contribute to your health.

Some people have allergic reactions to certain foods, including fruits. If you have mild food allergies, you may want to sample a small amount of a new fruit and wait a day to see if you have any adverse reaction before deciding to incorporate it into your diet. For those known to have more severe food allergies, or if you are nursing or pregnant, you should consult with your doctor before eating something you have never tried before.

The most effective way for me to help you put all of this great information into action is to show you how easy it is to make superfruits a regular part of your diet. I make it even simpler by also giving you recipes. In Part III, you'll find lots of delicious smoothie recipes that use superfruits, along with recipes for breakfast, salads, sauces, seafood entrees, and, to top it off, desserts!

The Superfruit Challenge

Would you be willing to change your diet if you could increase your chances of living healthier and longer? Combine that with looking younger, lowering your body weight, and reducing your risk of getting cancer, cardiovascular disease, or diabetes. All these benefits plus passing along healthier eating and lifestyle practices to your children. Sound good?

Having superfruits regularly in your diet means you can bank these advantages on your side. The top twenty fruits not only have superior nutritional properties but also are enjoyable to eat, commonly available, and inexpensive to use every day, justifying them as mainstays for your diet.

This book is about putting the relevant knowledge from available scientific facts into everyday dietary practice to strengthen your health and improve your life. Of greatest importance is the value superfruits have for promoting lifelong healthy eating habits for you and your loved ones. Could anything be more important and yet so simple? Let's get started!

Superfruits for Long-Term Wellness

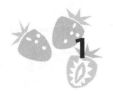

Essential Nutrients and Superfruit Signatures

A S WITH ANY PLANT or animal group, fruits vary in their characteristics, whether by shape, color, fragrance, taste, texture, or content of edible compounds. The fruits emphasized in this book are noteworthy for their appealing eating qualities and their variety of *essential nutrients* in higher concentrations than can be found in common fruits. In this chapter, I'll give you information about specific nutrients that distinguish certain fruits as truly *super*.

I'll also give you dietary reference intake (DRI) suggestions for the various nutrients discussed. DRI values are recommended for each nutrient by a panel of physicians and scientists affiliated with the Institute of Medicine, U.S. National Academy of Sciences. They represent daily target amounts of nutrient intake from the foods and beverages you consume. Each serving of food provides a proportion of DRI for a range of nutrients, making superfruits all the more valuable for your diet because they are "DRI-rich" fruits, both dense and diverse in nutrients. As DRI values are based mainly on a healthy body weight, amount per nutrient is generally higher in men than in women, with children having lower values.

Whether for meals or snacks, food and beverage intake should have a goal of getting the *maximum nutrient density* per serving, preferably from whole foods. This is why I focus on superfruits. By definition, they are super because of their high contents of nutrients essential for health!

Superfruit Signatures

When a given superfruit has a specific nutrient feature that makes it exceptional among other plant foods, I call this a "superfruit signature." Since we're talking about many nutrients in this chapter, there may be more than one signature that highlights a superfruit. Interpret "signature" as a general guide, because it is used only to help distinguish one fruit from another. The four signatures I cite are all in high amounts in top-rated superfruits:

1. Dietary prebiotic fiber (a *macro*nutrient needed in gram quantities)
2. Vitamin C (a *micro*nutrient needed only in milligram quantities)
3. Carotenoids (orange-yellow pigments, some of which are converted into vitamin A following digestion; they are a group of phytochemicals; the amounts needed are unknown)
4. Polyphenols (red-tan, blue-purple-black pigments; they are also a group of phytochemicals with undefined daily requirements)

FRUITS CONTAINING ALL FOUR SUPERFRUIT SIGNATURES IN HIGH AMOUNTS

A differentiating characteristic among superfruits is that only a select few are endowed with high amounts of all the superfruit signatures: (1) antioxidant vitamins A (from provitamin A carotenoids) and C, (2) prebiotic fiber, (3) mixed carotenoids, and (4) mixed polyphenols. Here are the best of the best for nutrient and phytochemical content:

▷ mango   ▷ orange

▷ red guava   ▷ seaberry

▷ dried goji (wolfberry)   ▷ papaya

Macronutrients

Expressed in gram (g) quantities for daily intake, macronutrients are relatively high-content food components that provide calories for energy, growth, cell activities throughout the body, or storage as fat. Macronu-

---

trients can be viewed as the true energy components of foods you eat, furnishing calories for your daily activities.

They differ from micronutrients by the quantities required: according to nutritional guidelines, daily macronutrient intake for an adult should include 130 grams of carbohydrates, about 50 grams of protein, 40 grams of fat, and 30 grams of fiber. All of the macronutrients featured in the following sections are considered essential for health and are present in all plant foods and superfruits in different amounts.

Carbohydrates, Proteins, and Fats

All plant foods and superfruits contain carbohydrates, proteins, and fats. Here is a quick overview of why plants contain them, what they mean, and how consuming them in superfruits allows us to benefit from them.

Carbohydrates are the most abundant major class of matter in plants. Plants use carbohydrates mainly for energy to support photosynthesis, growth, and the generation of structural components. All superfruits contain carbohydrates in forms we can taste—such as the natural sugars making fruits sweet—or experience by other sensory qualities such as texture, as in the crunch of an apple.

Proteins are made of amino acids arranged in chains joined by bonds that distinguish them as peptides. Proteins are essential parts of all plants and animals, participating in every process of cell structure and function. Some proteins are important for cell communication, immune responses, and life cycle. Proteins are also necessary in your diet, because the body cannot synthesize all the amino acids required for proteins to build cells, so you must obtain essential amino acids from proteins in your foods. Among superfruits particularly excellent as sources of amino acids and proteins are fig, goji, kiwifruit, seaberry, and guava.

Although the words *fats*, *lipids*, and *oils* are all used to refer to fats generally, *fats* usually refer to solid oils at normal room temperature, while *oils* refer to liquid fats, and *lipids* are a broader term for all. This category of molecules is important for many forms of life, serving both structural and metabolic functions, making it an important part of your diet as well. Examples of fats in edible plants, especially their seeds, are mono- and polyunsaturated ("heart-healthy") oils from peanuts, soybeans, sunflowers, sesame seeds, olives, and canola. Two superfruits, seaberry and açaí, are unusual in that they contain oil within their berry pulp, and several superfruits have edible seeds containing rich amounts of heart-healthy oils, including figs, red grapes, kiwifruits, blackcurrants, raspberries, and blackberries.

Dietary Fiber

Dietary fiber deserves special discussion because it is a "signature" nutrient of superfruits and because it has an important range of health benefits not often appreciated by the public. So, let's shine some light on dietary fiber—especially the kinds found in certain superfruits.

Plant fibers include natural components such as polysaccharides, gums, pectins, and inulins (prebiotic soluble fibers) as well as cellulose and lignans (insoluble fibers). These two kinds of fiber—soluble and insoluble—are in all plant foods. Soluble fiber is known as *viscous* or *prebiotic* fiber for, respectively, how it forms a watery gel in the upper digestive tract and becomes a food source for the billions of good bacteria in the colon of the lower digestive tract. Insoluble fiber does not become involved in any active digestive process but rather absorbs water and passes through the digestive system.

As end products of the normal colonic fermentation of the prebiotic fiber contained in superfruits, short-chain fatty acids contribute numerous physiological effects that promote health. For example:

► Aiding in insulin secretion and glucose absorption, possibly benefiting people with diabetes
► Providing nourishment to cells lining the lower intestine
► Reducing synthesis and absorption of cholesterol
► Stimulating immune defenses
► Increasing acidity of the lower digestive tract, which may inhibit formation of cancerous polyps

Fiber is necessary for your diet beyond its familiar function in maintaining regularity. The broader significance of prebiotic soluble fibers from superfruits, whole grains, and many vegetables is well recognized in science; in fact, four health claims for lowering the risk of cancer and cardiovascular diseases have been issued by the FDA.

By eating foods rich in these prebiotics, you also support your natural bacteria that promote digestive health. Take better care of your digestive health by increasing the amounts of prebiotic-rich foods such as super-fruits in your diet.

SCIENCE BEHIND IT

Many years of research have convinced the FDA that diets rich in pre-biotic fiber—such as polysaccharides from whole grains, including oats, barley, and psyllium—are effective for lowering levels of blood choles-terol and therefore may deter the onset of associated cardiovascular diseases and certain types of cancer. Rich in polysaccharides, super-fruits such as dried plums (prunes), oranges, raspberries, blackberries, figs, dates, açaí, mangoes, and goji berries (wolfberries) are notable for exceptional prebiotic fiber value.

Micronutrients

Micronutrients are an array of vitamins, minerals, omega fats, and plant sterols known from scientific studies to impart health values. Micronutrients are essential to your diet but only in amounts measured by the milligram (one thousandth of a gram, mg) or microgram (one millionth of a gram, mcg). They are defined as "essential" mainly because they can be obtained only from food, and if they are absent from your diet over long periods, you can develop a mild illness that can worsen if the nutrient absence persists. Superfruits, by definition, are especially rich in essential micronutrients, so simply by eating meals and snacks that include superfruits, you make these micronutrients work for you from day to day in supporting your health. Paying attention to micro-nutrient content during shopping and meal preparation is a valuable dietary practice over life.

Here are specific micronutrients particularly dense in superfruits:

- ▶ Vitamins A (from provitamin A carotenoids), C, and E—a group of antioxidants referred to as the "ACE" vitamins
- ▶ B vitamins
- ▶ Dietary minerals
- ▶ Sterols
- ▶ Omega fats

Antioxidant Vitamins A, C, and E

One valuable lesson about diets passed from generation to generation is that fruits are good food sources of vitamins. Thus, when it comes to superfruits, we expect more—and we get it. Let's have a closer look at this powerful group of ACE vitamins.

MYTH BUSTER

Many manufactured superfruit juices have been processed so extensively that the natural antioxidant ACE vitamins are completely absent, even if the product is advertised as an "antioxidant superfruit juice." Double—or even triple—pasteurizing is the main reason for vitamin loss. Check the Nutrition Facts panel on such products to see if ACE vitamin contents are at good-to-high percentages of the daily values.

Vitamin A. Vitamin A is a generic term representing several related retinyl chemicals with vitamin properties. Deficiency of vitamin A in your diet can lead to impaired night and sunlight vision, delayed wound healing, skin diseases such as eczema, abnormal skeletal development in children, and increased risk of infection, particularly of respiratory or viral origin.

Fruits and other foods do not actually contain vitamin A; rather, a group of the orange-yellow pigments called carotenoids, such as beta-carotene and beta-cryptoxanthin, are converted into vitamin A in the body.

Medical research on vitamin A has been extensive over the past fifty years, with more than three thousand publications cited in the U.S.

National Library of Medicine, the world's largest database of medical literature. Some of the most convincing research leads for vitamin A show clinical effectiveness against the following conditions:

▶ Progressive blindness in elderly people (also known as age-related macular degeneration, or AMD)
▶ Cancers of the prostate, skin, lung, blood, and lymphatic system
▶ Chronic inflammation, as in long-term osteoarthritis
▶ Pneumonia
▶ Measles
▶ Wrinkles, dermatitis, acne, and skin aging

Vitamin A carotenoids are especially important for healthy eyes and skin and for immune protection against infections. Superfruits that are excellent sources of vitamin A carotenoids include those with orange or yellow pulp such as mangoes, papayas, oranges, goji berries, gold kiwifruits, cherries, red guavas, and seaberries.

DIETARY REFERENCE INTAKE FOR VITAMIN A
The current DRI is 700 (women) to 900 (men) mcg, which is the equivalent of 2,333 to 3,000 international units (IU). For packaged goods, look on the Nutrition Facts panel for vitamin A content higher than 10 percent DV (daily value), and look on the ingredients list as well for a carotenoid provitamin A source—such as one of the superfruits.

Vitamin C. Vitamin C is the body's universal protector. As a water-soluble antioxidant, it locates in the body everywhere water compartments exist outside and inside cells. Also, cell elements and other vitamins associated with fat, such as vitamins A and E, are particularly dependent on vitamin C for protection against oxygen free radicals that may damage DNA and cell structure.

Vitamin C's main purpose in the body is to preserve iron for the hundreds of enzymes that depend on this essential mineral for their roles in metabolism. Even in small amounts, vitamin C has powerful antioxidant functions in body cells. It protects proteins, DNA, fats, carbohydrates, and other vitamins from reactive oxygen radicals, which are produced continuously by both normal metabolism and exposure to smoke, ultraviolet irradiation, and environmental pollutants. Among foods especially rich in vitamin C are color-rich superfruits such as oranges, kiwifruits, blackcurrants, strawberries, goji berries (wolfberries), seaberries, guavas, and mangoes.

DIETARY REFERENCE INTAKE FOR VITAMIN C
In adults, the DRI is generally stated as 75 (women) to 90 mg (men) per day, although other recent research indicates that *two to four times these levels* would be desirable and attainable by using supplements or eating superfruits and vegetables. One of the world's expert research centers on vitamin C, the Linus Pauling Institute at Oregon State University, recommends 400 mg per day, particularly for seniors, whose defenses against disease may weaken with aging.

Such an important vitamin for human health has attracted considerable research interest, as represented by some forty-one thousand medical research titles listed by the National Library of Medicine over the past century. Scientists usually first detect the importance of a nutrient to health by observing how diseases start and are sustained. In that light, here are a few leads from research regarding conditions against which vitamin C may act as an antidisease agent:

▶ Progressive blindness in elderly people
▶ Cardiovascular diseases, such as atherosclerosis and hypertension
▶ Onset mechanisms for cancers
▶ Chronic inflammation, as in long-term osteoarthritis
▶ Anemia
▶ Osteoporosis
▶ Neurodegenerative disorders such as Alzheimer's disease and Parkinson's disease

Vitamin E. Rather than a single substance, vitamin E is actually a family of eight antioxidants. The most nutritionally significant vitamin E is called *d-alpha-tocopherol*. Many superfruits contain d-alpha-tocopherol, especially those with pulp oils, such as seaberry and açaí, and those with edible seeds, such as figs, kiwifruits, red grapes, strawberries, raspberries, and blackberries.

Vitamin E may be the body's strongest antioxidant for protecting cell membranes and therefore is an essential guardian of sensitive cell functions. It is sometimes called the cell's "lightning rod" for its ability to neutralize reactive oxygen species. Other functions of vitamin E include facilitation of normal cell-to-cell communication and protective roles against nerve pain and dry or injured skin. Given such a wide number of organ functions, it's easy to see that this vitamin is crucial for health.

Convincing research leads for vitamin E show clinical effectiveness against the following conditions:

▶ A variety of cardiovascular diseases, especially atherosclerosis
▶ Various cancers
▶ Diabetes
▶ Chronic inflammation, as in arthritis
▶ Lung diseases such as asthma and those associated with smoking
▶ Impaired bone growth, healing and osteoporosis
▶ Neurological disorders such as impaired memory, balance, or coordination
▶ Neurodegenerative disorders such as Alzheimer's disease
▶ All disorders of oxidative stress, such as premature aging, bacterial infections, and gastric ulcers

DIETARY REFERENCE INTAKE FOR VITAMIN E
For adult women and men, the DRI is 15 mg per day, or 22.5 IU.

B Vitamins

There are eight B vitamins, all of which are involved in biochemical energy reactions at the cell level. Most superfruits contain high natural amounts of B vitamins, including B_1 (also called thiamine), B_2 (riboflavin), B_3 (niacin), B_5 (pantothenic acid), B_6 (pyridoxine), B_7 (biotin), B_9 (folic acid, or folate), and B_{12} (cyanocobalamin).

Dietary Minerals

The essential dietary minerals are imperative for good health and are easily obtained by eating whole superfruits and vegetables. The amounts of each mineral contained vary across superfruits but generally rate as good to excellent (more than 10 percent of daily value) for all.

Essential to bone health throughout life, *calcium* and *phosphorus* also have diverse other roles in human physiology, such as in the functioning of muscle cells, receptors for neural transmission, and energy processes in cells.

Varied roles in human cell functions involve fourteen other dietary minerals necessary for health. Most of these are in good to high levels in superfruits: *chloride*, for production of hydrochloric acid in the stomach and cellular pumps; *cobalt*, as a cofactor for vitamin B_{12}; *copper*, as a cofactor for numerous enzymes, including those essential for cellular respiration and metabolism; *iodine*, for synthesis of the hormone thyroxine; *iron*, for many enzymes and proteins, notably hemoglobin, which is the blood carrier of oxygen; *magnesium*, for energy-regulating enzymes; *manganese*, a cofactor in antioxidant enzyme functions; *molybdenum*, a cofactor for numerous enzymes; nickel, a urease enzyme cofactor; *potassium*, a systemic electrolyte and ion channel regulator with sodium; *selenium*, a cofactor essential to activity of antioxidant enzymes; *sodium*, a systemic electrolyte and ion channel regulator with potassium; *sulfur*, a cofactor for amino acid metabolism; and *zinc*, which is involved extensively in enzyme functions.

Each of these minerals is designated as *essential*, which can be interpreted both as the essential way in which they are involved in minute functions of human cells and as essential that we obtain them through foods, since our bodies do not synthesize minerals. A true superfruit should have both diversity and density of many essential nutrients, including minerals. Across the board, the top twenty superfruits provide excellent content of the sixteen minerals listed.

Phytosterols

Phytosterols are a group of plant chemicals called steroid alcohols (sterols), indicating that they have chemical structures like steroids that dissolve in lipid layers as easily as alcohol does. In the plant, sterols serve as a vehicle for communication between cells and for supporting anatomical structure.

Of nutritional interest, sterols are handled similarly to cholesterol and thus compete with it during synthesis (causing less cholesterol to be made) and transport from the digestive tract and blood into tissues (causing less cholesterol to be absorbed and deposited and therefore more to be excreted). Because dietary phytosterols lower blood cholesterol levels, they have been designated by the FDA as valuable nutritional components.

A 2004 clinical study at the University of California–Davis demonstrated that only 2 grams of phytosterol intake per day from drinking a fortified orange juice reduced blood low-density lipoprotein (LDL) cholesterol levels by 12 percent over just two months! Numerous other consumer products now contain phytosterols; examples are margarine, multivitamins, soy and rice milk, dairy products, bread, and granola bars. Look for these products and try to involve them in your diet, even if your LDL cholesterol level is normal.

Some superfruits have exceptional natural amounts of phytosterols in their skins, pulp, and edible seeds. Açaí berries, dried goji berries (wolfberries), and seaberries are examples of rich sources, but all whole superfruits would contain some, especially those having edible seeds (see Appendix B for more information).

DIETARY REFERENCE INTAKE FOR PHYTOSTEROLS
While a DRI for phytosterols is not yet officially established, ongoing research indicates that around 1.5 to 2 g per day is effective for reducing blood LDL cholesterol levels in adults. The FDA and Institute of Medicine are currently evaluating phytosterol research to assign a recommended intake level.

Omega Fats

Among the nutrient newcomers approved by science and the FDA just within the past few years, dietary omega-3 fats are now appreciated as essential for growth; maintenance of cell structure, particularly in the nervous system; and reducing the risk of cardiovascular disorders such as atherosclerosis, thrombosis, and coronary artery disease. Accordingly, the omega fats, which are polyunsaturated fatty acids (PUFAs) called docosahexaenoic acid (DHA) and eicosapentaenoic acid (EPA), are now accepted generally as a new and essential nutrient category.

Although most are easily obtained by eating cold-water ocean fish such as salmon, omega-3 fats can also be consumed through a plant-derived omega-3 oil called alpha-linolenic acid (ALA), which is found in some superfruit pulps, including açaí and seaberry, and in nearly all edible superfruit seeds, including those of the fig, red grape, goji, kiwifruit, blackcurrant, raspberry, and blackberry. Combining a meal of salmon with nuts, seeds, or superfruits with edible seeds would be an ideal way to assure good intake of omega fats.

Superfruit Signatures: A Summary

To help assure that you have a foundation of the high-content nutrients contained in most superfruits, let's summarize superfruit signatures:

► **Fiber.** Diets rich in dietary fiber, especially prebiotic fiber, have broad physiological benefits, including decreased blood levels of cholesterol and lowered risk of several types of cancer and coronary artery disease. The top superfruit sources of fiber are mangoes, figs, oranges, strawberries, the *Rubus* berries (raspberries, blackberries, boysenberries), goji berries (wolfberries), kiwifruits, dates, açaí berries (as a puree or pulp), seaberries, and dried plums (prunes).

► **Vitamin C.** The universal antioxidant, vitamin C has diverse roles in health, especially for maintaining skin and for connective tissue repair, along with eye, bone, teeth, and gum health. Except for processed or dried fruits in which the vitamin C content is reduced, all of the twenty superfruits are good to excellent sources of vitamin C, especially in their fresh form. Dried, frozen, and processed superfruits will have lower vitamin C content.

▶ **Carotenoids and Polyphenols.** Although not considered nutrients per se, these phytochemicals are highly diversified in chemical structure, are naturally abundant in plants as pigments, and are variably present in every superfruit. In the lab test tube, carotenoids and polyphenols are also antioxidants, possibly providing this role in the body. While science is still searching for better details, most experts agree that pigment-rich foods have general importance for health. Remember that phytochemical pigments give fruits their color! Also, vitamin A from carotenoids is a fat-soluble antioxidant stored for rapid-deployment defenses in the smallest lipid compartments of cells. Especially important for healthy eyes and skin and for immune protection against infections, the carotenoid-rich provitamin A superfruits are mangoes, papayas, oranges and other citrus fruits, goji berries, gold kiwifruits, cherries, red guavas, and seaberries. Even red or blue-black superfruits, such as cranberries, red raspberries, blueberries, blackcurrants, or blackberries, have carotenoids, but these are stored in seeds.

The central message from this chapter is that you should think of superfruits as exceptional sources of nutrients proved by science as essential for maintaining health. That said, superfruits are better known by the public for their phytochemical compounds such as carotenoid and polyphenol pigments. In the next chapter, I'll tell you about how phytochemicals are related to potential health and antidisease effects—a compelling but complex topic still being unraveled by scientists.

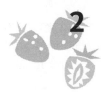

Superfruit Phytochemicals and the Health Value of Colors

THE POWER OF SUPERFRUITS exists mainly in their established natural nutrients but also is exhibited in other natural compounds, called phytochemicals. Among nature's astounding variety, phytochemicals comprise thousands of different compounds, including the pigments that give fruits their bright colors. Think of the wonderful red luster of a fresh strawberry: that crimson color comes from phytochemical pigments called anthocyanins, which hold potential value for health.

In each edible plant or fruit, there are dozens, if not hundreds, of phytochemicals with benefits that may transfer to you through a fruit's color and other potential health properties.

It's no coincidence that you've likely seen several health messages from respected groups such as the National Cancer Institute, Centers for Disease Control and Prevention, American Heart Association, and various government or other health organizations recommending that you eat five to ten servings of *colorful* fruits and vegetables daily. On this subject, four operative terms need to be understood:

▶ **Phytochemicals.** Plant scientists believe that there are more than eight thousand individual phytochemicals in nature! Medical scientists continue to analyze which ones may aid human health.
▶ **Pigment power.** Pigments giving fruits their colors are believed to have significant promise as health agents.

31

- ▶ **Functional foods.** Some foods are believed to have potential health-promoting and/or disease-preventing properties beyond just the basic nutrients. Superfruits are among these functional foods.
- ▶ **The Color Code.** A practical shopping and meal-planning guide has been created based on plant food colors and promising health effects. As superfruits are colorful foods, let's make use of this simple, practical guide!

Common Phytochemicals Found in Superfruits

Phytochemicals are natural, plant-derived chemicals that give fruits not only their color but also other qualities, such as fragrance, taste, or sourness. All components of a plant, including all known nutrients that we appreciate for their food value, are phytochemicals, but not all phytochemicals are nutrients!

Phytochemicals are produced mainly for defense of the seeds, the part of the plant that will assure the plant's regeneration. New research is examining a select few fruit phytochemicals for their potential health benefits to humans. Maybe you've heard about some of these tongue twisters:

- ▶ **Carotenoids.** The provitamin A compound beta-carotene, lycopene (abundant in tomatoes, pink grapefruit, and watermelons), and compounds called xanthophylls are all examples of carotenoids. Among the xanthophylls are lutein and zeaxanthin, about which you might have heard in the media concerning their health values for the eyes. Both serving as pigments in the human retina, lutein and zeaxanthin can be obtained easily by using orange or yellow superfruits in your diet.
- ▶ **Polyphenols.** Also called phenolic acids or phenolics, polyphenols are the parent class of several thousand compounds having similar chemical structure. Here is a list of the principal polyphenols to keep in mind for superfruits:
  - ▪ **Resveratrol**—a member of the plant defensive compounds called alexins
  - ▪ **Flavonoids**—a subfamily category of similar polyphenols

- **Anthocyanins**—a subfamily of flavonoids, the primary pigment group giving plant foods and flowers their colors of blue-purple-black or red-tan
- **Proanthocyanidins**—the parent compounds of anthocyanins, abundant in grape seeds and cranberries
- **Quercetin**—a flavonoid under research for potential actions against cancer and other diseases
- **Ellagitannins**—a class of bitter-tasting polyphenols comprising ellagic acid and tannin under research for various biological effects
- **Punicalagins**—a group of ellagitannins specifically found in pomegranate juice
- **Xanthones**—a type of defensive polyphenol often extracted from plant rinds for use as insecticides, but under research as potential antidisease agents

Carotenoid Pigments

Let's take a closer look at carotenoid phytochemicals. Fruits and vegetables that are red, orange, yellow, or green contain carotenoids. These pigments associated with the vivid colors of tomatoes, carrots, and corn may wield powerful benefits for our health. Food carotenoids have two characteristics of particular health value to us. First, once digested and circulated in the body, they tend to dissolve best in lipids and therefore are concentrated in fatty parts of human cells such as the membranes and nuclear envelopes, as well as the sheaths of nerves close to critical functions of these cell components. Second, carotenoids have a chemical structure effective for neutralizing potential damage caused by oxygen radicals.

In ongoing laboratory research on animals, carotenoids have been linked to health benefits associated with the following conditions:

- ► Eye diseases
- ► Cardiovascular diseases
- ► Cancer
- ► Skin diseases such as psoriasis
- ► Inflammation
- ► Viral infections

Polyphenols

Active medical research indicates that polyphenols from various plant foods hold the promise to favorably impact human health. For example, there is preliminary evidence that polyphenols act against these major threats:

- ▶ Metabolic syndrome and obesity
- ▶ Osteoporosis and bone loss
- ▶ Cancer of various types
- ▶ Premature aging
- ▶ Cardiovascular diseases
- ▶ Age-related eye diseases

We must be cautious about what conclusions we draw from new research on polyphenols in relation to superfruits. The polyphenol class as a whole is a highly productive research topic in food and medical science. While scientists are continually adding to what we know about the possible impact of these plant compounds on human health, we need to be wary about the use of unconfirmed results for marketing by manufacturers eager to have a competitive edge in selling superfruit products. This practice unfortunately leads to false claims of effectiveness and to their acceptance by consumers as fact when actually the research is too premature to warrant conclusions about health benefits.

Phytochemical Guidelines

We can gain a view of how phytochemicals are defined in nutrition guidelines by reviewing the following excerpt from the position statement of the American Dietetic Association:

> In addition to the nutrients that are involved in normal metabolic activity, foods contain components that may provide additional health benefits. These food components (generally referred to as *phytochemicals*) are derived from naturally occurring ingredients and are actively being investigated for their health-promoting potential.
>
> These phytochemicals and/or health-preserving elements are present in a number of the foods that we often eat, especially fruits, vegetables, grains, legumes, and seeds, and in a number of less frequently consumed

foods such as licorice, soy, and green tea. In addition, functional foods, which can be defined as any modified food or food ingredient that may provide a health benefit beyond the traditional nutrients it contains, are being developed and subjected to scientific evaluation. In recent years, the number of functional foods that have potential benefits for health has grown tremendously. Scientific evidence is accumulating to support the role of phytochemicals and functional foods in the prevention and treatment of disease.

Dozens of phytochemicals are under study for their potential effects in humans. The benefits may be similar to the roles they are known to perform for the plant itself. In plants, phytochemicals defend against disease invaders, ultraviolet exposure, bacteria, viruses, fungi, DNA and cell damage, and destructive free radicals.

One fact from nutrition research on phytochemicals is clear: eating a whole food (usually its edible portions of pulp, skin, and occasionally seeds) guarantees taking in as many intact phytochemicals and nutrients as possible. Once inside our bodies, the *nutrient* complement of the whole fruit may act together with phytochemicals, a process some health professionals call *nutritional synergy*.

Leading Edges of Research on Superfruit Phytochemicals

Superfruit phytochemicals are being researched intensively for their potential health benefits to people. These phytochemicals are being studied for possible preventive qualities against certain diseases.

Resveratrol

Among all the current superfruit research going on, no individual phytochemical has ignited as much research intensity as resveratrol. Resveratrol is present not only in red grapes and wine but also in the skins of superfruits such as blackcurrants, blueberries, and strawberries.

Resveratrol acts as a kind of universal immune guard against environmental pathogens. It creates a defensive front line of protection on the fruit skin, vine epidermis, and leaves against attack by pests and diseases. If you eat fruits rich in resveratrol, you are already practicing part of a functional-food diet because of this phytochemical's research promise for benefiting human health!

In current research, resveratrol is being examined as a potential preventive agent for what many scientists consider the pinnacle challenge of modern health issues—aging. Certain to involve innumerable onset factors, aging not only is a natural process that can occur gracefully but also is a condition in which many people become vulnerable to major diseases. Postponing aging would be interesting for some folks; deterring or preventing age-related diseases among elderly people would be welcomed by everyone.

SCIENCE BEHIND IT
The research excitement about resveratrol began with a study in 2003 at Harvard University indicating that resveratrol mimicked effects of calorie restriction in yeast cells, extending their longevity by 70 percent. Its main target in the body appears to be an enzyme called sirtuin, which, in addition to its properties as an antiaging molecule, can lower blood sugar levels in mice bred to have diabetes and obesity.

As studies on resveratrol progress, evidence is gathering that it enhances biological defenses against aging by doing the following:

► Inhibiting inflammation
► Regulating anticlotting factors that affect blood coagulation and thrombosis
► Deterring onset of cancer
► Enhancing fat metabolism
► Reversing cognitive deterioration
► Improving working memory
► Delaying or preventing onset of Alzheimer's disease
► Delaying or preventing progression of vascular disease
► Regulating factors that control blood vessel tone
► Inhibiting oxidative stress/reactive oxygen species

Cardiovascular Diseases

Cardiovascular diseases are a major cause of death in developed countries, making prevention a priority for public health policy. Research evidence over years has shown that cardiovascular diseases can be managed and even prevented by healthful eating practices involving a resveratrol-enriched diet of whole plant foods such as offered by superfruits. For more than fifty years, research has shown that a healthful, active lifestyle combined with the dietary benefit of high fruit and vegetable intake may lower blood lipid levels, blood pressure, and risk of coronary heart disease and stroke.

Large-scale population studies of a whole-food Mediterranean diet (see also Part III and Appendix D for references) supplemented with fruits reduced the risk of cardiovascular diseases by about 15 percent compared with people having lower whole-food and fruit intakes. Among 125,000 people who consumed eight or more servings of fruits and vegetables daily, there was a 20 percent lower risk of developing cardiovascular diseases compared with those consuming fewer than three servings. Eating just one extra fruit or vegetable daily decreased risk by an additional 4 percent.

Any number of nutrients and phytochemicals may contribute to the protective effects of superfruits in your diet, including increased amounts of mono- and polyunsaturated fats, the antioxidant ACE vitamins, B vitamins, potassium and several other minerals, prebiotic fiber, carotenoids, and polyphenols, as well as resveratrol.

Cancers

Results of experimental and clinical studies indicate that eating a diet rich in fruits and vegetables decreases the risk of developing various types of cancer, particularly those of the lungs and digestive tract. Experimentally, evidence for the anticancer effect of a whole-food diet has come from research previously discussed and from studies of freeze-dried black raspberries, a species of raspberry especially rich in anthocyanins shown to inhibit cancer in the rat esophagus by 30 to 60 percent and in the rat colon by nearly 80 percent. Black raspberries are a practical research tool and a promising therapeutic source, as they contain dense contents of these specific phytochemicals.

In other laboratory studies, anthocyanins, tannins, or other polyphenols from red grapes, black or red raspberries, blackberries, strawberries, cranberries, blueberries, goji berries (wolfberries), açaí berries, or pomegranates were shown to inhibit promotion and growth of premalignant cancer cells by the following specific mechanisms:

- ▶ Accelerating tumor cell turnover, called apoptosis, effectively making the cancer cells die faster
- ▶ Reducing inflammatory mediators involved in tumor onset mechanisms
- ▶ Inhibiting new blood vessel growth that nourishes tumors
- ▶ Minimizing cancer-induced DNA damage of normal cells
- ▶ Turning off genes involved with proliferation, apoptosis, and inflammation

Also, by studying anthocyanins from superfruits, scientists have discovered a possible *synergistic* anticancer activity with other polyphenols such as tannins, proanthocyanidins, and flavonols.

Metabolic Syndrome, Obesity, and Diabetes

Clinicians project that during the next thirty to fifty years 40 percent of Americans will develop metabolic syndrome, the majority being seniors but also an alarming increased number of children. Metabolic syndrome is the co-occurrence of several known disease risk factors, including insulin resistance, obesity, high blood cholesterol, and hypertension, conditions that are interrelated and share the same onset mediators, mechanisms, and pathways. People with these pathologies are at a heightened risk for developing cardiovascular diseases and diabetes.

Such gloomy forecasts have ignited new research efforts and advisory programs to educate the public about dietary and lifestyle modifications to prevent and control these conditions. The promising benefits of dietary resveratrol were discussed earlier in this section. Consumption of nutrient-dense, high-fiber foods—as in a Mediterranean diet supplemented with extra fruit servings—is recommended by many nutritional and medical experts.

Experimental properties of phytochemicals with potential health value in this area include the following:

▶ Inhibiting growth of individual fat cells
▶ Suppressing the rapid rise in blood glucose and insulin levels following a meal
▶ Stimulating expression of immune cells called cytokines, affecting fat cell growth and multiple immune functions
▶ Altering gene sensitivity controlling fat metabolism, causing fat cells to limit their activity and growth
▶ Deterring development of overall obesity

Osteoporosis

Higher intakes of fruits, specifically superfruits and certain vegetables, are also associated with improved bone mineral density and reduced bone loss in both men and women. Clinical trial results indicate that a diet rich in fruits and vegetables preserves bone health. Other studies link bone health to superfruit phytochemicals such as carotenoids, flavonoids, quercetin, and vitamin C. For example, in the Framingham Osteoporosis Study conducted over four years at Tufts University, in Boston, loss of bone mineral density in hundreds of elderly women and men was inversely related to intake of dietary carotenoids—a phytochemical found in superfruits!

Age-Related Vision Loss and Macular Degeneration

Degeneration of the retinal macula of the eye is the leading cause of blindness in people over age sixty-five in the United States. Lutein and zeaxanthin are dietary carotenoids found in relatively high concentrations in the retina, where they may inhibit damage caused by direct sunlight. Studies at the University of Hohenheim, in Germany, and the Hong Kong Polytechnic University showed that the Chinese superfruit goji (wolfberry) contains both zeaxanthin and lutein in significant amounts, as well as beta-carotene, other nutrients, and polyphenols that may act together to support vision health.

A diet rich in carotenoid fruits and vegetables, especially those containing lutein and zeaxanthin—as found in some superfruits, including mango, guava, and seaberry—may lower the risk of developing age-related macular degeneration (AMD), a condition of deteriorating eyesight. According to the ongoing Age-Related Eye Disease Study (AREDS) by the U.S. National Eye Institute, examining thousands of seniors, higher dietary intake of lutein and zeaxanthin is associated with decreased incidence of AMD.

Aging and Neurodegenerative Diseases

Although it is not yet clear whether a diet rich in fruits and vegetables will decrease the risk of neurodegenerative diseases such as Alzheimer's or Parkinson's in humans, recent studies at Tufts University using rat models indicate that diets high in blueberries, strawberries, and blackberries may be protective against these diseases.

The Tufts research shows that a fruit diet including polyphenols from dark berries appears to positively impact learning and memory in aged rats, possibly due to a direct effect on aging neurons, cell-to-cell signaling, and neuronal calcium buffering.

Color Code, Pigment Power, and Superfruits on the Front Lines of Research

As you now know, fruit phytochemicals such as carotenoids and polyphenols associated with the color of superfruits have potential health properties—this fact is the premise of the Color Code, first presented years ago in separate books by Drs. David Heber and Jim Joseph (see complete references in Appendix D). Colors from nature's palette of pigments represent a simple way to keep superfruits in mind for your daily meals and snacks! Later on, I'll show you how superfruits and the Color Code can be an easy visual guide to shopping for healthy meal planning.

The list of fascinating compounds contained within nature's most complex fruit treasures is so long that the accompanying table can illustrate only a few superfruit phytochemicals currently under study, by way of example. We owe it to ourselves to be aware of the path that scientists are taking to unveil all relevant properties of superfruits and their wondrous compounds.

While this research is unfolding, wouldn't it be wise to begin the practice of eating a nutrient- and phytochemical-rich superfruits diet *now*? Diseases are not inevitable and may actually be prevented by adopting sound dietary habits based on superfruits with pigment power and the Color Code.

RESEARCH PROGRESS OF SUPERFRUIT PHYTOCHEMICALS TOWARD HEALTH CLAIMS

Color code	Phytochemical	Typical superfruit or plant food source(s)	Potential disease intervention(s)
red-tan; blue-purple-black	resveratrol	red grapes	cancer, metabolic syndrome, Alzheimer's disease
red-tan; blue-purple-black	mixed polyphenols	citrus fruits	cardiovascular
red-tan	anthocyanins	cranberries	cardiovascular
red-tan; blue-purple-black	proanthocyanidins	cranberries, grape seed extracts	urinary tract and other bacterial infections, cardiovascular
red-tan; blue-purple-black	flavonoids	dark berries	inflammation, diabetes, cancer, cardiovascular, blood clotting
blue-purple-black	quercetin	dark berries	asthma, cancer, diabetes
orange-yellow; green	beta-carotene	mixed fruits, vegetables	various diseases
orange-yellow	lutein, zeaxanthin	citrus fruits, marigold petals, goji berries	age-related eye diseases
orange-yellow	citrus flavonoids—hesperidin, naringin, luteolin	oranges and other citrus fruits	bone disorders

All these phytochemicals are in advanced human research for clinical study in step 4 of the research pyramid (see Introduction).

Functional Foods and Superfruit Phytochemicals

"Let food be thy medicine and medicine be thy food," stated Hippocrates 2,500 years ago, a statement that was never more apparent than it is now. From physicians and nutritionists to governments and consumers, there is increasing interest in learning how specific foods and their nutrients can improve and sustain health. An example of a functional food is calcium-fortified orange juice, which contains added calcium to enhance bone health, cell activities in many organs, and other roles in normal body functions. Another example is soy milk fortified with multiple nutrients.

Let's think about the red grape, one of my top twenty recommended superfruits. Red grapes are good sources of resveratrol, which is well advanced in medical research as a potential antiaging and antidiabetes compound. Red grapes, especially very dark varieties such as Concord, are also among the richest natural sources of anthocyanin pigments, giving these grapes their dark purple color. Remember that phytochemicals such as anthocyanins are being extensively researched for numerous possible health properties. If anthocyanins are eventually proved to contribute health benefits, then red grapes and red wines can be seen as more "functional" than their white grape counterparts.

What could be easier for giving yourself the best possible health maintenance from nutrients, the disease-fighting properties of phytochemicals, and the potential antiaging advantages of resveratrol than simply eating more delicious and colorful superfruits? In the next chapter, you'll see nature's top twenty superfruits up close—ten berry species and ten tree fruits.

The Superfruits

Nature's Top Twenty Superfruits

A s discussed in Part I, superfruits have extraordinary nutrient and phytochemical quality. They exhibit more density and diversity of these attributes than other fruits. For a fruit to be truly "super," it must also convince scientists around the world to study and publish their findings regarding its exceptional promise for health-promoting properties, such as by lowering disease risk or slowing the aging process.

I'll give you a list of fruits that truly are super, ranking them in order of nature's most nutrient-packed fruits. I'll also share with you the salient research behind them and explain why these great-tasting and some-times exotic fruits can be a boost to lifelong wellness. I hope that you'll be encouraged to incorporate these specific fruits in a well-balanced diet and excited about the significant promise superfruits hold to enhance your health.

Superfruit Score: How the Top Twenty Were Picked

The twenty fruits that are the most nutrient dense and most promising in regard to their health properties were selected from a set of five criteria, each having a high score of 5:

► **Nutrient diversity and density.** A truly super fruit should contain many nutrients, with several in particularly rich amounts for achieving the dietary reference intake (also called daily value) in a single serving.

► **Phytochemical diversity and density.** Phytochemicals (*phyto* meaning "plant") are natural plant compounds whose properties are not yet understood but have promise for being important to human health. (Examples are carotenoids and polyphenols, as outlined in Part I.)

► **Basic research intensity.** Usually well before the public hears about a new scientific fact, investigators have been on the trail for years doing laboratory research—called "basic" for work in test tubes and experimental animals. As this is occurring now for the top twenty superfruits, I have tracked superfruit basic research to give you a glimpse of what scientists are learning. A simple index of this progress is the number of publications in reputable journals to represent the breadth, intensity, and duration of research inquiry on each fruit.

► **Clinical research intensity.** This indicator shows how close science is to proving that a superfruit used regularly in one's diet could lead to better human ("clinical") health or disease resistance.

► **Popularity.** Because this is certainly the most important qualifier for anyone to call a fruit "super," I wanted fruits on my top twenty list to be appealing to many consumers. For superfruits to be adopted generally, people should be able to quickly recognize them when shopping and regularly use them in a healthy diet. Popularity factors include sensory appeal, such as appearance, fragrance, color, and taste; ease and versatility of use; reliability of supply; and cost-effectiveness. Some consumers are concerned about calorie intake so a ratio of nutrient value/sugar content to estimate caloric burden may be important when choosing fruits for your diet.

Once each fruit is scored, the tally is what I call the Superfruit Score, providing a basis for ranking the twenty fruits. A fruit complete in all five criteria would truly be "super," but few fruits actually achieve high scores for all five across the board.

Mango (*Mangifera indica*) INDIAN SUBCONTINENT, SOUTHEAST ASIA, MEXICO

SUPERFRUIT SNAPSHOT

Nutrient Content: high in protein, prebiotic fiber, antioxidant vitamins A and C, B vitamins, dietary minerals

Phytochemical Content: high in carotenoids (alpha- and beta-carotene, beta-cryptoxanthin, lutein, violaxanthin), polyphenols (quercetin, gallic acid, gallotannins, rhamnetin, cyanidin and xanthone glycosides, including mangiferin, mainly in skin)

Color Code: red-tan, orange-yellow, green (mango has numerous cultivars, or cultivated varieties, of different colors)

The fruit that tops my list is the mango. Among the world's most widely cultivated and most popular fruits, the mango originated in the Indian subcontinent and Asia. Mangoes account for about half of all tropical fruits produced in the world. With United Nations estimates of world-wide production at more than thirty-three million tons annually, mango is one of the most widely consumed among the top twenty superfruits. Delicious in their various tastes, colors, and sizes, mangoes come in some fifty cultivars. Four of the most popular are the Palmer (red, elongated), Tommy Atkins (red-tan or orange-yellow-green, plump), and Alphonso and Ataulfo (both yellow, kidney-shaped); all are rich in flavor. The mango has a firm, fragrant, and visually appealing internal pulp, usually golden and like a cantaloupe in texture, flavor, and color, although with a denser fruit body and less moisture.

Why Mangoes Are Super

The mango is particularly high in superfruit signatures—prebiotic dietary fiber, vitamin C, carotenoids and polyphenols. The mango also contains a broad range of essential nutrients at good to excellent levels for dietary reference intake, especially the dietary antioxidants vitamin A (from carotenoids) and vitamin C. Vitamin B_6 (pyridoxine), other B vitamins, essential minerals, amino acids, and omega fats are at good levels. As discussed in Part I, many of these essential nutrients are required for health because they are involved in diverse biological processes in the body. Among all superfruits, mango provides the most comprehensive nutrition, popularity of taste, and versatility of uses across many world regions.

The mango's edible peel and pulp contain both types of pigments—carotenoids and polyphenols. As many as twenty-five different carotenoids have been isolated from mango pulp, the densest content of which was beta-carotene (a provitamin A compound), accounting for the yellow-orange flesh of most mango species. As health-promoting prebiotic fiber, polysaccharides (long-chain sugar molecules natural to plants) are also a major mango constituent of value for your diet. The peel and pulp include carotenoids (provitamin A beta-carotene, lutein, and alpha-carotene as possible antioxidants) and polyphenols, lupeol and a unique phytochemical called mangiferin, a specific mango extract under study for its antidisease properties.

Although mango skin offers extra nutritional benefit of dietary fiber, carotenoids, and polyphenols, not everyone enjoys its more fibrous texture, and the majority of users would likely exclude it. However, if steamed or in a stir fry, the skin will soften and become less chewy. Also, rarely, some people may be sensitive to a natural chemical in mango skin called urushiol that can cause skin blisters.

Research Behind Mangoes

The subject of more than 750 research publications since the 1930s, mangoes have been a continual mind spring of scientific knowledge for isolating potential therapeutics and healthful dietary agents. The range of research on mangoes covers nearly every area of nutrition and common human diseases.

Over the past decade, Cuban and Spanish scientists have examined several disease models using Vimang, a blend of extracts from different parts of the mango fruit and tree. Vimang is a concoction rich in mangiferin and has experimental effects against certain types of allergens, inflammatory substances, and pain. In one 2008 experiment, Vimang improved memory and other signs of neurological function in rats. In addition, a mangiferin-enriched compound made in India from mango tree leaves showed antibiotic activity against specific dental bacteria in human subjects, indicating that toothbrushing with mango extracts could benefit oral hygiene.

Also of research interest is mango lupeol, a natural terpene demonstrating an array of biological activities against inflammation, arthritis, DNA damage, and malaria in both test-tube and animal experiments. Interest in developing lupeol-based anticancer agents has led to discovery of numerous highly active derivatives exhibiting significant potencies and therapeutic indications across different types of cancer. Although more research is needed to clarify cancer-preventive compounds, extracts of mango and its juice were shown to inhibit cancer cells in laboratory experiments.

Mangoes in the Research Pyramid

One practical outcome of research on a fruit is its widespread application as a food for alleviating diseases associated with malnutrition. Particularly in impoverished western Africa, mango is a practical food source of nutrients, especially provitamin A carotenoids, dietary fiber, and vitamin C—each essential for relief from childhood malnutrition and recognized by international organizations assisting famine regions of Africa. Greenhouse solar dryers, for example, are being constructed to prolong mango storage and recover edible by-products from processing to treat the widespread malnutrition. Among all superfruits, mango has the most extensive global infrastructure as a comprehensive source for combating such nutritional deficiencies.

Get Mangoes into Your Diet!

Offering rich flavor, fresh whole mango varieties are worth several tests of your own to find a favorite to use often in fruit dishes, smoothies, and garnishes (explore the website of the National Mango Board, mango.org/en.aspx). The juice quality is high, and the beverage has always been a favorite in the Caribbean region. My favorite daily use? Oatmeal with fresh mango pieces and vanilla yogurt. A bowl of this to start your day gives a nutrient-rich boost to get you all the way to noon. Dried mango slices are increasingly seen in grocery store bulk bins or packaged fruits, providing opportunity to involve this superb fruit for snacks on the go. While fresh, of course, is best when it comes to preserving essential nutrient content, the mango is also enjoyable and nutritious as frozen or dried fruit, 100 percent pure juice, and a flavor increasingly popular in common products. Just a third of a whole mango is one serving.

 MANGO SUPERFRUIT SCORE
Superfruit Score: 23/25
Rank Among 20 Superfruits: 1st
Nutrient Content: 5/5
Phytochemical Content: 5/5
Medical Research Activity: 4/5
Position in Research Pyramid: 4/5
Popularity: 5/5

Fig (*Ficus carica*, **numerous species) MIDDLE EAST, MEDITERRANEAN BASIN, WIDESPREAD TROPICAL ORIGIN AND DISTRIBUTION**

SUPERFRUIT SNAPSHOT
Nutrient Content: high in protein, prebiotic fiber, antioxidant A-C-E vitamins, B vitamins, dietary minerals
Phytochemical Content: high in carotenoids (beta-carotene), polyphenols (anthocyanins)
Color Code: black, red-tan

If Mother Nature had a vote for her ultimate superfruit, this would probably be it. After all, didn't she stock the promised land with figs? Given their distribution across the world's tropics, home to dense populations, figs are among the most exploited of tree fruits. They are a healthy staple of diets in every corner of the world, but they are not always used for food; countless folk medicine remedies in the form of poultices are used to treat various minor skin and internal disorders in African, Middle Eastern, and Asian countries.

When you look at the nutrient content of figs, the overall significance of this fruit as a high-impact food source becomes instantly clear. Manufacturers seem to recognize this fact as well, as products containing figs can be found as dried whole fruit (the preferred format), nutrition bars, smoothies, yogurt, cereals, fruit leathers, and—the best known of all—cookies: the Fig Newton!

Why Figs Are Super

Figs are a convenient single-food source broad in nutrient content, having exceptional amounts of insoluble and prebiotic dietary fiber, essential dietary minerals, and an unsaturated omega-6 fat, linoleic acid. Essential vitamins A (from carotenoids), B, and K are also present in high densities in the fig. These vitamins have an array of uses in the body—from antioxidant and metabolic roles to participation in blood coagulation and vascular function—that together support cardiovascular health.

Figs also provide a source of caloric energy from carbohydrates and a boost of micronutrients, including an unsaturated omega-3 fat, alpha-linolenic acid, in their numerous chewable seeds.

As for phytochemicals, figs are complex, containing numerous carotenoids, especially the provitamin A beta-carotene, and a variety of polyphenols. The skin of figs contains more fiber, phytochemicals, and antioxidant activity than the pulp, with antioxidant capacity proportional to the content of anthocyanins. As a rule of thumb, darker fig varieties, such as the black mission fig, have a greater content of polyphenols than lighter-colored varieties. If possible, use the darker variety for more nutritional and phytochemical value. Dried figs are chewier, more portable, and generally better liked than fresh figs.

Research Behind Figs

Given the phytochemical complexity of figs, this fruit is a treasure trove for basic research. Currently, there are potential applications for figs and its extracts against cancer, microbial and viral infections, pain, skin diseases, sun exposure, cardiovascular and digestive disorders, metabolic syndrome, and nutritional deficiencies, to cite only a partial list. As many of these diseases could have a common origin from inflammatory mechanisms, recent research on the potential health properties of figs has focused on their antioxidant and anti-inflammatory effects.

Figs in the Research Pyramid

Similar to the mango, the fig is a food regarded by nutritional scientists as a nutrient-rich, common resource that may help alleviate malnutrition in undeveloped countries. This practical application justifies its position high in the research pyramid. Also a staple of the Mediterranean diet—a dietary pattern widely regarded as the healthiest—figs are favored for their potential role in reducing the morbid trend of metabolic syndrome affecting millions of people in developed countries.

Studies in Europe are under way involving figs in controlled diets to test for specific health benefits in people with cardiovascular disease, obesity, diabetes, or chronic inflammation.

Get Figs into Your Diet!

If you began your childhood enjoying Fig Newtons, as I did, then this fruit likely has been a favorite for life. Now I find that the whole dried fruit couldn't be handier at lunch or as a snack food. Choosing the darkest, softest ones, such as black mission, assures optimal nutrition combined with eating pleasure and potential phytochemical richness. The tiny seeds are actually an enjoyable crunch, well worth the effort to release their extra nutrient value in the form of vitamin E, minerals, and polyunsaturated omega fats.

Dried figs are a nutritious, convenient superfruit, perfect for snacking—offering a healthy source of calories to meet the day's energy needs as well as the potential benefits of phytochemical diversity. Just four figs equal one fruit serving.

FIG SUPERFRUIT SCORE
Superfruit Score: 22/25
Rank Among 20 Superfruits: 2nd (tied with orange)
Nutrient Content: 5/5
Phytochemical Content: 5/5
Medical Research Activity: 4/5
Position in Research Pyramid: 3/5
Popularity: 5/5

Orange (*Citrus sinensis*) SOUTHEAST ASIA, BRAZIL, UNITED STATES

SUPERFRUIT SNAPSHOT
Nutrient Content: high in protein, prebiotic fiber, antioxidant A-C-E vitamins, B vitamins, dietary minerals
Phytochemical Content: high in carotenoids (beta-cryptoxanthin, beta-carotene, lycopene in red varieties), polyphenols (hesperidin, anthocyanins)
Color Code: orange-yellow, red—"blood" pulp varieties

Often taken for granted because they are so common, the varieties of orange—navel, Valencia, Persian, blood, cara cara, tangerine, mandarin—offer diversity in tastes and applications among consumer food and beverage products. Did you know that orange pulp and its pith—the white, fleshy material surrounding and interwoven among segments—is an excellent source of dietary fiber? The fiber value comes from pectins and polysaccharides—prebiotic fibers—which contribute toward lowering the risk of cancer and reducing blood cholesterol levels.

Right there in front of us all along, the common orange is a fantastic whole-food superfruit.

 FUN FACT!
Traded on the New York Stock Exchange, orange juice is the only superfruit product that is a commodity in global trade.

Why Oranges Are Super

Are we guilty of overlooking and underappreciating this universally popular fruit? The delicious pulp of a raw orange contributes all the major signatures of a superfruit: high levels of vitamins A (as beta-carotene) and C, prebiotic and insoluble fiber, and carotenoid and polyphenol pigments. Oranges are also rich in calcium, several B vitamins, potassium, and iron and contain good levels of other essential nutrients that support general health. The edible peel (for garnish, condiments, marmalades, and desserts) contains an abundance of superfruit signatures—vitamins A and C, prebiotic fiber, carotenoids, and polyphenols. As a popular flavor and fragrance, this superfruit is the whole package!

Let's not ignore a familiar item at the breakfast table: 100 percent pure orange juice—and it *should* be there as a reliable nutrient kick to start the day. OJ gives you an infusion of vitamins A (via carotenoids), B, and C, along with other micronutrients at good levels. I like it with lots of pulp, knowing that those tiny morsels are surrounded by membranes of plant fiber, packing an extra prebiotic fiber advantage!

Research Behind Oranges

Variants of oranges by cultivation have proved that levels of phytochemical pigments differ according to color. For example, the blood orange and the red-fleshed cara cara are richer in anthocyanins and lycopene than a typical navel orange. All oranges contain polyphenols, anthocyanins, other flavonoids such as hesperidin (present in the pulp but denser in the peel), and hydroxycinnamic and citric acids, which give the fruit its tangy flavor. Many of these compounds are well on their way in research regarding their anti-inflammatory and antioxidant mechanisms that may better define potential disease fighters.

Who would have thought that the orange peel is also packed with a variety of citrus phytochemicals? Orange peel is typically used for zest, essential oil fragrances, and marmalades, but it actually contains a host of complex, flavorful phytochemicals. One peel extract, d-limonene, is under active research as a potential gastric acid neutralizing agent that may relieve heartburn and gastroesophageal reflux. D-limonene also has well-established anticancer activity in laboratory studies.

Oranges in the Research Pyramid

Orange constituents have been studied extensively in various disease models for their ability to inhibit inflammation, allergies, blood cholesterol levels, cardiovascular disorders, and cancer.

Both orange juice and oranges as a whole food are involved in current and recently concluded clinical trials, indicating that this fruit as a source of candidate antidisease agents has reached the top of the research pyramid. At the University Hospital of Bordeaux in France, investigators have devoted particular attention to the potential benefit of orange juice carotenoids, flavonoids, and micronutrients in affecting vascular function and blood cholesterol levels among subjects with elevated blood lipids. The research evidence is almost complete. Eating this fruit combines the known beneficial effects of dietary fiber and vitamin C with the anticipated benefits from its carotenoid and polyphenol phytochemicals, which may lower the risk of major diseases such as cancer and cardiovascular disorders.

Get Oranges into Your Diet!

Few fruits have a more generally appealing taste than the orange. Its popularity as a juice alone qualifies it for the highest rank available, but other products in which you'll find it include granola and whole-fruit bars, marmalade, and as an ingredient of yogurts, beverages, and juice blends.

A near-perfect natural health food, a raw whole orange embodies abundant nutrient and phytochemical diversity in a package you can open yourself! Rich in fiber (include the white pith) and vitamin C, a juicy, delicious whole orange makes for an easy way to get the main superfruit signatures—fiber, antioxidant A-C-E vitamins, carotenoids, and polyphenols. Just one small navel orange equals one fruit serving.

Don't discard your orange peels! They have a variety of uses. For example, you can make and store zest for flavorings and dessert toppings by scraping the peel with a zester, knife, or peeler. You can also chop the peel and add small pieces to your favorite jams, jellies, and syrups of any flavor for extra citrus zestiness! Remember that there are a lot of valuable citrus phytochemicals in the orange peel alone.

ORANGE SUPERFRUIT SCORE
Superfruit Score: 22/25
Rank Among 20 Superfruits: 2nd (tied with fig)
Nutrient Content: 5/5
Phytochemical Content: 4/5
Medical Research Activity: 4/5
Position in Research Pyramid: 4/5
Popularity: 5/5

Strawberry (*Fragaria vesca, Fragaria ananassa*)
CALIFORNIA, EUROPE

SUPERFRUIT SNAPSHOT
Nutrient Content: high in prebiotic fiber, antioxidant vitamin C, dietary
   minerals
Phytochemical Content: high in polyphenols (skin and pulp anthocyanins, particularly pelargonidin, and ellagic acid and ellagitannins in
   the achenes)
Color Code: red

As a superfruit, strawberries score well on all five criteria—but no one
would need scientific evidence to think of this fruit as super. Everyone
seems to love strawberries just for the eating experience and the many
pleasures of their color, fragrance, and taste.

Production volumes of strawberries for the grocery market also indicate a rising demand for this first berry of summer. For example, the
export volume of strawberries from California has doubled just over the
past few years.

FUN FACT!
Strawberries are in the same family as the rose plant family called *Rosaceae*, as are other superfruits such as blackberries and raspberries.

Why Strawberries Are Super

Strawberries are outstanding sources of vitamin C and dietary fiber, two
significant superfruit signatures. Having a wide range of other micronutrients, strawberries are notable especially for high levels of the dietary
mineral manganese, plus good contents of other micronutrients. Strawberries also are rich in diverse polyphenols and contain two compounds
strongly related to health benefits—phytosterols (cholesterol-lowering
effects) and resveratrol (possible antiaging and antidiabetic effects).
Recognized by the many yellow achenes (which appear to be seeds but

are actually the true fruit!), strawberries provide significant content of achene omega-3 and -6 fats. The popularity of the strawberry along with its diverse and rich nutrient content make this a near-perfect superfruit!

Research Behind Strawberries

The rich red color of strawberries comes from numerous phytochemicals of the polyphenol family and its major subgroup, flavonoids, which are densely found in strawberries. One flavonoid class in particular, anthocyanins, accounts for most of the red pigmentation of strawberries, but also present are ellagic acid, ellagitannins, catechins, and cinnamic acid, each having significant health research interest. In preliminary laboratory tests, these strawberry polyphenols are showing evidence that they may lower the risk of inflammation, cancer, and cardiovascular diseases.

An interesting study performed by Oregon scientists showed that the strawberry's yellow achenes comprise only 1 percent of the berry's weight but contribute up to 14 percent of the total phenolic strength of the whole berry! Phytochemical polyphenols identified in strawberry achenes were ellagic acid and two anthocyanins, pelargonidin and cyanidin, each a strong antioxidant in laboratory studies. Moreover, once digested and distributed in the human body, these polyphenols are thought to have other subtle roles that involve modifying enzyme activity, receptor sensitivity, or gene activation, some of which could have bearing on the course of diseases. Whether applicable to prevention of or recovery from disease mechanisms, this theory is an active research topic in the quest to understand how berries and other superfruits may inhibit chronic inflammation and cancer onset.

SCIENCE BEHIND IT

In scientific terminology regarding anthocyanins, the compound is expressed as a sugar, such as *cyanidin-3-glycoside*. Across the top twenty superfruits, including strawberry, red grape, cranberry, blueberry, raspberry, blackberry, blackcurrant, and açaí (all red, blue, or black berries), cyanidin is among the most prevalent in content and most widely researched of all anthocyanins. Cyanidin research may eventually be a key to unlock the mystery of how superfruits in the diet favorably affect cell functions in health and diseases.

Strawberries in the Research Pyramid

Since 1929 when the first report on strawberries was recorded, PubMed (the database of medical literature from the U.S. National Library of Medicine) citations total more than one thousand individual research studies on strawberries, with nearly 10 percent of the total just in 2008, reflecting recent growth of research intensity. Strawberries have a compelling health story that features emerging research evidence of their ability to lower the risk of various diseases: thrombosis (susceptibility to blood clots and embolism); high blood cholesterol and associated vascular disease, including coronary artery (heart) disease; chronic inflammation; initiation, progression, and proliferation of several types of cancers; various symptoms of premature aging (e.g., skin disorders, visual decline); gastrointestinal reflux disease; immune insufficiencies; and viral, bacterial, microbial, parasitic, and fungal infections.

At the University of Toronto, studies examining specific dietary effects related to lowering blood cholesterol show that people adhere to a prescribed diet more faithfully and have reduced cholesterol levels when strawberries are included in daily meals. Such diets incorporate fruits, vegetables, soy products, prebiotic fiber (such as from oatmeal), plant sterols, and nuts. Look for references to this work in Appendix D and more information in Part III on the "Portfolio" diet

By this evidence, strawberry research has climbed up the research pyramid to the top, requiring only proof of efficacy in human trials to indicate a specific health benefit that satisfies FDA approval criteria.

Get Strawberries into Your Diet!

Bursting with one of the most popular fruit tastes, strawberries are favored around the world, easily ranking them at the pinnacle of superfruit flavors. Could strawberry be the world's most popular berry? Maybe that's too limiting, as it could be the world's most "fun" and popular food of all. Think of the many varied strawberry products: jam and preserve, syrup and topping, granola bar, cereal, pie, ice cream, smoothie, wine, fruit leather, gum, and the famous strawberry milk shake, shortcake, chocolate-covered berry, and daiquiri. It even has a party named after it—the strawberry social! The dense red pigmentation indicates the presence of additional polyphenols and correlates with the fruit's highest vitamin C and sugar contents, making strawberries especially good just for eating fresh—brighter fruits with red internal pulp tend to be better eating. Just five strawberries equal one fruit serving.

STRAWBERRY SUPERFRUIT SCORE
Superfruit Score: 20/25
Rank Among 20 Superfruits: 4th
Nutrient Content: 4/5
Phytochemical Content: 3/5
Medical Research Activity: 4/5
Position in Research Pyramid: 4/5
Popularity: 5/5

Goji (wolfberry, *Lycium barbarum*) CHINA

SUPERFRUIT SNAPSHOT
Nutrient Content: high in prebiotic fiber (polysaccharides), antioxidant vitamins A (from beta-carotene) and C, dietary minerals, phytosterols
Phytochemical Content: high in carotenoids (zeaxanthin, beta-cryptoxanthin, beta-carotene, lycopene), polyphenols (anthocyanins, ellagic acid)
Color Code: red, orange-yellow

The wolfberry, commonly called the goji, grows primarily in the region of northern China called Ningxia. Its reputation in China was built on the numerous applications it has had in traditional medicine for maintaining vision even into old age. How wise the ancient Chinese herbalists were, as goji berries are rich in at least twelve nutrients important for eye health! Nutrient dense, available mostly as dried fruit but also as a delectable, tomato-like juice versatile for flavoring blends, goji has gained popularity rapidly in Western countries just in the past few years and was named by industry journalists as "superfruit of the year" for 2008.

FUN FACT!
"Goji" was popularized first in the United States by a juice marketed as though the berries came from high in the Tibetan Himalaya Mountains, giving the product an aura of rare pristine origin. In actuality, the origin of goji berries is the central China regions of the Yellow River valley, more than a thousand miles from the Himalayas.

Why Goji Berries Are Super

Goji is one of nature's special food gifts, a fruit laden with diverse nutrients, some of which approach or exceed 100 percent daily value from a 100-gram serving. Among nutrients in which it is rich are vitamins A (from beta-carotene) and C, riboflavin (vitamin B_2), and five dietary minerals—copper, magnesium, potassium, selenium, and zinc—all of which are involved in a host of enzyme functions that maintain health. This fact is one key to goji's possible contribution to overall well-being: just by having a rich diversity of essential nutrients, goji can influence most biological processes, all of which depend on enzymes, which in turn rely on mineral cofactors.

Also significant in goji is its rich content of polysaccharides, which are high in macronutrient value as prebiotic fiber, providing a host of potential health benefits, such as the capability of lowering blood cholesterol and reducing cancer risk.

Research Behind Goji Berries

Typical of many members of the botanical plant family *Solanaceae*, which also includes the tomato, eggplant, and pepper, goji is phytochemically rich, characterized by having both major classes of pigments—carotenoids and polyphenols, identified in laboratory research as having antidisease mechanisms. Goji appears to be one of the richest plant sources of the carotenoid zeaxanthin (closely related in chemical structure to the better-known lutein), which is taken up selectively by the human retina as a pigment, apparently for filtering intense sunlight. When localized in tissue, zeaxanthin and lutein appear as orange-yellow pigments, giving a small region of the human retina called the macula lutea the only such pigmentation in the body. The fruit contains cholesterol-lowering phytosterols and good levels in its seeds of vitamin E and omega-3 and -6 fatty acids, which are important to cardiovascular and brain health.

Goji Berries in the Research Pyramid

In scientific literature, the goji is referred to by its original name, wolfberry. As of early 2009, this fruit, having centuries of legendary use and decades of research interest in China, has still not stimulated significant enthusiasm among scientists outside Asia. In Asian laboratories, the berry's constituents are under an extensive range of basic research, including potential applications against cancer; loss of vision with aging; cardiovascular, neurological, and inflammatory diseases; and immune disorders. A research group in Hong Kong has focused especially on the fruit's potential antiaging effects, providing preliminary evidence for the inhibition of beta-amyloid toxicity in neuronal cell cultures (a laboratory model for Alzheimer's disease) and the protection of retinal cells in experimental glaucoma. Discovering the specific compounds involved in these effects and the mechanisms by which they prevent eye diseases may reveal key information regarding how goji berries and similar natural products can support lifelong eye health.

Get Goji Berries into Your Diet!

Dried goji berries are the most popular and most common product format. Having the consistency of low-moisture raisins, they may be an acquired taste for some consumers to appreciate the unfamiliar blend of tomato-nut-cranberry flavors! Goji berry pieces are being used more often as ingredients in nutrition bars and cereals. Just thirty dried goji berries equal one fruit serving.

Goji is also available as an orange-red, sweet, rich juice with fruity, tomato-like flavors, making it a novel ingredient and color for blending with more ordinary juices. In specialty stores and on Internet sites, you'll mostly find diluted juice products in which goji has been combined with at least one other fruit juice, such as apple or grape. A few companies do provide the nutrient-rich goji juice by itself either in whole form or concentrated, with only the water removed. These whole juices are as close as we can get a beverage to the optimum natural wholesomeness of goji berries.

GOJI SUPERFRUIT SCORE
Superfruit Score: 19/25
Rank Among 20 Superfruits: 5th (tied with red grape)
Nutrient Content: 5/5
Phytochemical Content: 3/5
Medical Research Activity: 4/5
Position in Research Pyramid: 3/5
Popularity: 4/5

Red Grape (*Vitis vinifera*) NATIVE TO EUROPE; GLOBAL IN TEMPERATE AND SEMITROPICAL REGIONS

SUPERFRUIT SNAPSHOT
Nutrient Content: high in antioxidant vitamin C, dietary minerals
Phytochemical Content: high in polyphenols, including resveratrol and the richest content of anthocyanins yet described for fruits
Color Code: red-purple-black

Grapes are certainly one of the more popular fresh and processed superfruits. Favored by every cuisine and culture, they grow readily in temperate regions as far north as British Columbia's Okanagan valley and northern Germany, and as far south as Peru, South Africa, and Australia.

Why emphasize *red* grape as a superfruit? Only red, rather than white or green, is included because its skin color derives from additional phytochemical pigments, mostly anthocyanins, some of which have promise as health agents. Standing tall among these red grape phytochemicals is the research superstar, resveratrol. (Remember our discussion about resveratrol in Part I?) Resveratrol is a polyphenol with exciting promise as a protective compound against premature aging, diabetes, and cancer.

Why Red Grapes Are Super

In value of actual nutrients, red and green grapes differ little, having a broad range of low to moderate levels of essential macro- and micronutrients. Both red and green grapes feature excellent contents of vitamins K and A (from carotenoids contained mainly in their seeds). Make it a point to select and chew grapes with seeds, for extra vitamin A, vitamin E, omega-3 and omega-6 fatty acids, and seed polyphenols called proanthocyanidins. These compounds may have numerous roles in maintenance of general health of the blood, skin, and brain, and in laboratory studies, grape seed proanthocyanidins inhibit cancer and inflammation mechanisms.

Research Behind Red Grapes

The scientific history of the red grape since 1881, when its first medical publication was recorded by PubMed, shows that attention has been directed to its phytochemicals mainly from the skins and seeds, both of which contain a greater diversity of compounds that may benefit health more than the pulp.

Of specific intense research interest for their exceptional anthocyanin and resveratrol contents are native American grape species with the thickest, darkest skins—the two most famous being Concord and muscadine. Both varieties yield exceptional contents of skin anthocyanins and resveratrol.

Notably, Concord grape juice in the diet has shown significant research progress for lowering blood cholesterol levels, inhibiting blood clots, reducing cancer onset, and improving physical performance and cognitive function in experimental animals. Consistent with this interpretation, Dr. Steve Talcott, a food scientist at Texas A&M University, and his colleagues published a 2009 study showing that the dense polyphenols in cabernet sauvignon and muscadine grapes could inhibit the amyloid protein deposits and neuropathology in a mouse model of Alzheimer's disease.

The human research with purple grape juice has been even more exciting, with promising results shown for lowering blood pressure and reducing the incidence of Alzheimer's disease in the Kame Project, a study of nearly two thousand elderly Japanese Americans in Washington state. The Kame Project results also indicate that moderate consumption of purple grape juice (just three or more servings per week) or red wine improved cognitive abilities—perhaps good evidence, after all, that red grapes and other anthocyanin-rich superfruits are indeed brain foods!

Red Grapes in the Research Pyramid

The grape is likely the most studied fruit, with more than four thousand medical research publications in the past 130 years. Interest in its many consumer products, including the health benefits of drinking wine, has increased the range of scientific inquiry. Current clinical research is evaluating potential health benefits of grape products related to aging and major diseases, including inflammation, several types of cancer, and cardiovascular diseases.

Owing to the importance of grapes in human diets and to the ascendance of promising phytochemicals such as resveratrol and anthocyanins in the research pyramid toward clinical trials, the red grape is the most intensively studied and most advanced superfruit in human research.

In a late 2008 review entitled "Grape Products and Cardiovascular Disease Risk Factors," two Spanish scientists summarized the last thirteen years of research progress in understanding how grapes in the diet may affect cardiovascular diseases. Most of the published studies examined specific mechanisms of grape phytochemicals or focused only on the suspected benefits of regular, moderate consumption of red wine. From review of seventy-five clinical trials, the authors showed that polyphenols, wine alcohol, and dietary fiber were the main favorable grape factors, producing major outcomes such as lower blood pressure, lower blood cholesterol, and evidence of improved vascular function.

Get Red Grapes into Your Diet!

Representing one of the world's most popular flavors, snacks, drinks, and garnishes, red grapes have no problem achieving the highest possible score in this category. Think of their many product forms and uses: fresh in an array of dark hues, dried (as raisins), jam, juice, and wine—to name a few. Grapes are also used for a multitude of flavors, fragrances, and colors. Explore the wonderful variety of red grape products to regularly add enjoyment and potential health benefits to your diet. Just fifteen grapes equal one fruit serving.

RED GRAPE SUPERFRUIT SCORE
Superfruit Score: 19/25
Rank Among 20 Superfruits: 5th (tied with goji)
Nutrient Content: 2/5
Phytochemical Content: 4/5
Medical Research Activity: 4/5
Position in Research Pyramid: 4/5
Popularity: 5/5

Cranberry (*Vaccinium macrocarpon*) UNITED STATES

SUPERFRUIT SNAPSHOT
Nutrient Content: high in prebiotic fiber, antioxidant vitamin C, dietary minerals
Phytochemical Content: high in polyphenols, including anthocyanins, proanthocyanidins, and ellagic acid
Color Code: red

As can be seen by their common genus name, *Vaccinium*, cranberries and blueberries are close botanical relatives and thus have similar physical characteristics and nutrient profiles. Wild or cultivated across the northern hemisphere, cranberries have been popularized by a red "juice cocktail" with a tangy taste and clean finish. They also are a traditional sauce or jelly side dish for winter holiday dinners and are gaining popularity as dried, sweetened fruit.

Why Cranberries Are Super

Cranberries contain most essential nutrients at good or low levels, as well as three with excellent daily value percentages—dietary fiber (mainly from skin), vitamin C, and manganese. In addition, cranberries have significant polyphenolic content, especially tannins; proanthocyanidins, mainly responsible for the characteristic tartness; and anthocyanins, the primary pigments for their crimson color. Through mechanisms that may involve anti-inflammatory, antibacterial, or antioxidant effects, all these polyphenols are under active research for their potential roles in lowering the risk of onset of numerous human diseases. Among the twenty superfruits, cranberries are near the top for intensity of research interest and progress up the research pyramid toward conclusion of human clinical trials.

Research Behind Cranberries

Among berries, the cranberry is the third-most studied (after grape and strawberry), being the subject over the past century of more than five hundred research reports on laboratory models of cancer, heart disease, inflammation, aging, and ulcers. Cranberries have been studied most extensively for the specific antibacterial properties of proanthocyanidins, which may inhibit adhesion of bacteria to epithelial tissues such as those of the urinary tract ("anti-adhesion" effects).

Among twenty-five clinical trials on cranberry juice or extracts in early 2009, half were investigating specifically these anti-adhesion/antibacterial effects. The largest, most advanced study is a series of related phase II clinical trials by the U.S. National Center for Complementary and Alternative Medicine of the National Institutes of Health involving 250 to 400 female patients in each study. This research is distinctive among superfruits in that it is related *not* to the hallmark of public interest in superfruits—antioxidant properties—but rather to antibacterial effects.

Recognized subjectively for sourness, cranberries have this flavor profile because of their richness in a variety of polyphenols (phenolic acids), which increase the acidity of the fruit. This characteristic is also the most probable health factor in cranberries, as phenolic acids may be the beneficial factor for inhibiting growth of urinary tract bacteria and of stomach bacteria (*Helicobacter pylori*) that cause the formation of peptic ulcers. Separate studies in 2008 by scientists in Japan, China, and Chile showed that regular consumption of cranberry juice inhibits *H. pylori* colonization in adults and children and, therefore, may be effective in preventing stomach infections and even some cancers.

Another noteworthy result of cranberry polyphenol research is the berries' possible use in oral health products such as mouthwash, dental floss, and toothpaste. Imagine that: a cranberry-infused and -flavored toothpaste or dental floss that actually kills bacteria in dental plaques. Brilliant!

Cranberries in the Research Pyramid

The cranberry research centered on the anti-adhesion and antibacterial effects obtained from regular juice consumption, which were discovered nearly fifty years ago, has led to a health claim allowance in France, and several clinical trials are under way in the United States. Although cranberry juice and tablet products are commonly taken to prevent urinary tract infections, an optimal effective dose has not been established, and the cranberry phytochemicals responsible for anti-adhesion properties are not yet defined precisely; proanthocyanidins are considered the leading candidate for effectiveness. Other current clinical trials aimed at determining potential benefits of cranberry juice include subjects with diabetes, cancer, cardiovascular diseases, and visual deficits associated with aging. Cranberries are an example of a fruit whose health-promoting potential was discovered at a relatively early time in modern science—the 1960s. Antimicrobial effects were found just from regularly drinking diluted juice, still a worthwhile reason for adding this juice to your diet.

Get Cranberries into Your Diet!

Cranberries require sweetening if used in fresh or frozen form, yielding tangy, slightly sour products that many people enjoy in sauces, compotes, jams, and syrups. What would Thanksgiving or Christmas dinner be without cranberry sauce, and why are we not dishing up this delicious sauce more frequently throughout the year? The common retail juice itself is eminently versatile, adding mild tartness that blends readily with other fruit juices and sauces. One fruit serving equals an eight-ounce glass of juice cocktail or about twenty-five dried berries—two easy ways to get this outstanding superfruit into your diet.

CRANBERRY SUPERFRUIT SCORE
Superfruit Score: 18/25
Rank Among 20 Superfruits: 7th (tied with kiwifruit)
Nutrient Content: 3/5
Phytochemical Content: 3/5
Medical Research Activity: 4/5
Position in Research Pyramid: 4/5
Popularity: 4/5

Kiwifruit (*Actinidia deliciosa*) CHINA, NEW ZEALAND

SUPERFRUIT SNAPSHOT
Nutrient Content: high in prebiotic fiber, antioxidant vitamins A (higher in the gold kiwi) and C, dietary minerals
Phytochemical Content: high in chlorophyll, carotenoids (beta-carotene, lutein), polyphenols (mixed flavonoids)
Color Code: green or gold

The kiwifruit is odd-shaped, having the form and size of a perfect egg covered in a fuzzy, dark green coat, which helps to preserve freshness and adds to its appeal. It's just the right size for frequent use as a fresh food. Grown in China for decades in Western obscurity, the kiwifruit became better known when horticultural expertise in New Zealand started contributing to the world's supply. New Zealand is now the world leader in kiwi production and has adopted this fruit as a national symbol.

New horticultural advances have made the once unique light green pulp a feature of a separate cultivar that is richer in carotenoids. Called the Zespri, it is identical in shape to the original green kiwi but features a gold color and a lighter, sweeter taste. Due to its increasing global popularity, the Zespri has rapidly become one of New Zealand's major export crops. Further breeding development by New Zealand horticulturalists in 2008 has led to a totally new kiwi with bright red pulp from enhanced anthocyanin content; it is yet to be named.

Why Kiwifruits Are Super

Similar to the case with figs, you cannot eat kiwi without encountering delightful little black seeds that add to the nutrition and enjoyable textures. Kiwi ranks near the top of all natural foods in vitamin C and fiber content and has excellent levels of potassium, omega-3 and omega-6 fatty acids, and vitamin E (abundant in the seeds). Although the skin is fuzzy—possibly deterring some users—it is an excellent source of dietary fiber and pigments. If you are fortunate to find the new hybrid gold kiwi, Zespri, take advantage of the extra nutrient values from the orange-yellow carotenoids and the contribution of beta-carotene to forming antioxidant vitamin A in the body.

Research Behind Kiwifruits

Kiwis are notable for having phenolics that impart a citruslike fresh taste to the fruit; chlorophyll, giving the green appearance; and carotenoids from the seeds and pulp in the gold Zespri. In the past few years, scientists have isolated the densest protein present in kiwis, named *kiwellin*, which appears to have promising activity for studies of immune response.

The results of laboratory tests using the gold kiwi, published by New Zealand scientists in early 2008, showed that immune biomarkers were increased in mice after twenty days of eating a puree of the gold kiwifruit. Ovalbumin, an immune stimulant, significantly increased blood levels of immune-response compounds and enhanced antigen-specific proliferation of cells in lymph fluid. These results indicate that gold kiwifruit can provide an antigen-specific immune response, possibly revealing a new type of functional food ingredient.

Other scientific interest surrounds a derivative of kiwellin called *kissper*, also an extract from kiwi. Kissper is a member of a new class of pore-forming peptides that influence cell membrane porosity having potential for biotechnology developments in drug delivery.

Kiwifruits in the Research Pyramid

The phytochemical complexity of kiwis has attracted scientific interest for the potential health effects involved, including laboratory studies to probe for activity against cancer, inflammation, diabetes, metabolic syndrome, microbial infections, and immune disorders.

Applied kiwi research, however, is still mainly in the discovery stage, with few animal studies and no clinical trials, placing kiwifruit in the bottom half of the research pyramid. However, this exceptional fruit is certain to be the subject of extensive research in the future.

Get Kiwis into Your Diet!

A fresh kiwi is one of the "funnest" fruits to eat due to its pleasant appearance, citrus taste, and unique mouth feel—a cool, refreshing sensation and seed crunchiness. More to the point, that fun comes with a rich content of all the superfruit signatures. The new gold Zespri has the look of something special, making it a dynamic addition to any fruit platter or garnish. Occasionally in grocery and bulk food stores, one can find kiwi juice or freeze-dried slices that extend the product's shelf life and portability. Just one kiwifruit equals one serving—making it easy to regularly include this nutrient treasure in your meals and snacks.

KIWIFRUIT SUPERFRUIT SCORE
Superfruit Score: 18/25
Rank Among 20 Superfruits: 7th (tied with cranberry)
Nutrient Content: 4/5
Phytochemical Content: 4/5
Medical Research Activity: 3/5
Position in Research Pyramid: 2/5
Popularity: 5/5

Papaya (*Carica papaya*) CENTRAL AMERICA, CARIBBEAN REGION, WORLDWIDE TROPICS

The papaya is one of those rare treats typically introduced to northern travelers visiting the tropics; afterward, its delicious features as a fresh fruit and juice remain in the memory forever.

One of the most widely used tropical fruits, the papaya is favored in its native countries for fresh eating, for juice, and as an ingredient in jellies, preserves, and cooked meals, including its young leaves, shoots, skin, and seeds. Papaya seeds in particular, which are bitter to eat raw, have intriguing medicinal properties that are exploited in traditional practices to treat infections from bacteria, amoebas, parasites, and fungi. More practically, the ground dried seeds are an interesting condiment alternative to pepper.

The papaya fruit yields a protein-digesting enzyme called papain, which is used in numerous industrial applications, including meat tenderizers, chewing gum, candies, and beer clarification. It is also used as a potential therapeutic in medicine, where it is being tested for treating skin conditions. Cosmetically, papain appears as an ingredient in shampoos and skin creams, some toothpastes as a whitener, and spa treatments.

In South America, the papaya (probably for its papain content) is used as a home remedy for jellyfish, bee, and wasp stings; mosquito and snake bites; and even stingray wounds (efficacy uncertain), for its ability to break down protein toxins in the venom. It is also an ingredient in some first aid creams and may be used as an enzymatic agent for treating infected skin wounds.

In the realm of superfruits high in nutrient content and with broad potential for contributing industrial advantages for consumers, papaya is a leader and among the most versatile.

Why Papayas Are Super

A particularly rich source of vitamins A (from beta-carotene) and C, papaya is also a standout in providing good levels of prebiotic fiber, potassium, B vitamins, and essential minerals. Although not generally considered palatable enough for chewing, the numerous black seeds of a papaya are an excellent source of micronutrients and omega fatty acids. The seeds also are loaded with phytochemicals, particularly isothiocyanates and glucosinolates, which are valued in vegetables such as broccoli and cauliflower (brassica sources).

Research Behind Papayas

As a primary carotenoid food source, papaya is an inviting subject for studying this pigment class and its contributions in relation to provitamin A compounds. Papaya also harbors other phytochemical secrets that are just being discovered, especially its value as a brassica chemical resource from seeds and pulp. There is a growing amount of research specifically on papain, which belongs to a group of plant enzymes found in the papaya. Scientists in Brazil showed that papain is involved in virtually every aspect of plant physiology and development. It plays a role in development, maturation, and aging of the plant; storage and mobilization of proteins; and response to environmental stress. Papain may be related to human enzymes involved in blood clotting, digestive processes, tumor development, and wound healing.

Papayas in the Research Pyramid

Studied in preclinical research for nearly ninety years, the papaya has produced a diverse literature totaling more than nine hundred reports to date. Its testing in antidisease models is highly diversified and includes inflammation, diabetes, and cancer, as well as viral, bacterial, parasitic, and cardiovascular diseases.

Papain has reached clinical trials for treating leg venous ulcers seen in severe diabetes. An experimental drug containing papain is being tested for safety in treating skin irritation, changes in wound debridement status, and use in possible skin grafts.

Remember that the fruit seeds are indeed more powerful in phytochemical content than the fruit itself. In a Nigerian study showing that air-dried papaya seeds were effective as dietary therapy for treating human intestinal parasites, the investigators proposed that eating papaya seeds offered a natural, harmless, simple, and inexpensive therapeutic benefit against intestinal parasititis in tropical communities.

Get Papayas into Your Diet!

During my first visit to the Bahamas in 1971, I was introduced to papayas through a preparation later to take the United States by storm—fruit smoothies. During a particularly hot noontime in Nassau, a street vendor, parked outside a hotel supplying electricity to his food blender, was making smoothies from papaya, pineapple juice, and vanilla ice cream, resulting in a refreshing, orange-yellow "slurpie" that satisfied the calorie demands for an afternoon of scuba diving. To this day on hot summer afternoons, that is still a favorite treat!

Papaya has a soft, moist orange-red pulp somewhat similar to that of a ripe peach but smoother; its skin is edible if cooked. Cut into chunks, papaya pulp is refreshing as a breakfast side dish and blends easily for smoothies, giving them a characteristic red-orange hue. Included last during preparation of a stir-fry, or lightly microwaved, it adds color, tropical taste, and high nutrient qualities to meals. Increasingly, American grocery stores and fruit stands stock papayas of different cultivars. Just a third of the whole fruit equals one fruit serving.

PAPAYA SUPERFRUIT SCORE
Superfruit Score: 17/25
Rank Among 20 Superfruits: 9th (tied with blueberry, cherry, red raspberry, and seaberry)
Nutrient Content: 4/5
Phytochemical Content: 3/5
Medical Research Activity: 4/5
Position in Research Pyramid: 3/5
Popularity: 3/5

Blueberry (*Vaccinium angustifolium*, *Vaccinium corymbosum*) CANADA, UNITED STATES

A public icon of health in recent years, blueberries, once grown only in Canada and the United States, have ratcheted up in popularity so extensively that global competition for the fresh market now includes such countries as Peru, Argentina, Mexico, and China. The increased supply from the southern hemisphere also means we can enjoy this fruit fresh or frozen year-round, making it an easy superfruit choice for adding to your shopping cart and freezer. After all, how many pure blue foods can you select from nature's palette of fruit colors? None as true blue as this one!

When you're purchasing the fresh produce, you will typically find two blueberry sizes, representing two distinct but related species: the smaller, pea-size, "low-bush" variety, which was cultivated from original wild plants of Atlantic Canada and northern forest understories; and the grape-size, American highbush species, which was developed specifically to yield larger fruit on taller bushes, making the crop easier to pick with mechanical harvesters.

Why Blueberries Are Super

What impresses about blueberry's nutrient profile is that it has a broad range. Almost all essential nutrients are present at low to good levels for achieving daily value percentages—similar to its close cousin, the cranberry. Three nutrients with excellent DV percentages are dietary fiber (mainly from the berry skin), vitamin C, and the essential mineral manganese. The main attraction of blueberries may be the skin's unique profile of blue-pigmented anthocyanins and resveratrol, two intensively researched scientific topics.

Research Behind Blueberries

Blueberries are notable for their anthocyanin content, which imparts the blue skin color, but they also contain other polyphenols with potential health value. For example, the proanthocyanidin compounds made famous by the success of cranberry juice as a possible antibacterial, anti-adhesion agent for relieving urinary tract infections also are present in blueberries. Blueberries or their phenolic extracts are being studied for potential roles in a variety of conditions affecting human health. Anthocyanins such as cyanidin and delphinidin glycosides are being investigated for their effects on aging, memory, physical performance, inflammation, cardiovascular, metabolic, and anticancer mechanisms.

Blueberries in the Research Pyramid

Topics for hundreds of medical research studies since its first appearance in medical literature in 1927, the blueberry is still stimulating investigation for its potential roles against inflammation, some types of cancer, osteoporosis, and cognitive decline with aging, among other maladies.

Blueberries have given rise to more than three hundred scientific studies in the past fifty years. However, for specific testing in human research against disease, progress has been slowed by the inability to isolate blueberry components active in the human body.

Also, in contrast to the case with some other superfruits, there is no leading consumer brand built just on blueberries—curious to me, because this fruit would have been my first pick to develop commercially as a superfruit—and therefore, no one company has stepped forward to finance the expensive series of basic and clinical research steps that might reveal blueberry's specific health benefits.

Blueberry research is still mostly in the bottom half of the research pyramid, but a few early-stage clinical trials involving either blueberries mixed with other fruits or blueberry juice are under way to determine potential effects on cardiovascular disease, inflammation, lung cancer in women, and cognitive decline during aging. Blueberries have been especially promising in rat studies of aging; in research done at Tufts University in Boston, diets supplemented with blueberry extracts showed ability to slow and even reverse age-related deficits in rats, perhaps due to the fruit's antioxidant and anti-inflammatory properties.

FUN FACT!
Blueberries are the official provincial fruit of Nova Scotia and are the state fruit of New Jersey! In the United States and Canada, July is designated as Blueberry Month.

Get Blueberries into Your Diet!

Featuring a widely popular color and taste for numerous culinary preparations from cereals to salads to desserts, blueberries are a commonly favored fruit. An excellent snack fresh by themselves, they are truly wonderful in pies, jams, smoothies, and syrups. Blueberries in oatmeal, cold breakfast cereal, and salads; as garnish for vegetable stir-fries and meat dishes; or just popped into your mouth as an on-the-go snack are delectable ways to keep this superfruit regularly in your diet! A mere quarter cup of blueberries equals one fruit serving.

SUPERFRUIT SCORE
Blueberry Superfruit Score: 17/25
Rank Among 20 Superfruits: 9th (tied with papaya, cherry, red raspberry, and seaberry)
Nutrient Content: 3/5
Phytochemical Content: 3/5
Medical Research Activity: 4/5
Position in Research Pyramid: 2/5
Popularity: 5/5

Sour or Sweet Cherry (*Prunus cerasus*—sour, *Prunus avium*—sweet) TEMPERATE ZONES OF NORTH AMERICA, EUROPE, ASIA

SUPERFRUIT SNAPSHOT
Nutrient Content: high in prebiotic fiber, antioxidant vitamins A (from moderate carotenoid content) and C, dietary minerals
Phytochemical Content: high in polyphenols (anthocyanins)
Color Code: red, dark purple; gold varieties

Demonstrated by the endless stream of consumer products containing the cherry taste, cherries are among the most popular fruits. Easy and even fun to eat, sweet cherries have more sugar content and a lower density of phenolic acids than tart (or sour) cherries. Otherwise, the two species, sweet and sour, are cousins within the rose plant family, *Rosa-*

ceae, so are related botanically to other superfruits—strawberry, red raspberry, and blackberry.

Sour cherries have a more sour taste profile than sweet cherries due to the higher content of polyphenols, including the color-rich pigment anthocyanins in their skins; there is also lower sugar content in the pulp and juice of sour cherries. Some sour species are a deep maroon color when ripe. Because of these superior chemical "defenses," while still on the tree, sour cherries are better able to repel pests and airborne diseases than sweet cherries. Also owing to the high anthocyanin content, sour cherries are promising dietary agents for reducing the risk of inflammation, pain, high blood lipid levels, cancer, and metabolic syndrome.

Why Cherries Are Super

The bright red-orange color of cherries tells us something about nutrients. There are provitamin A carotenoids, probably beta-carotene, in the fruit and also significant amounts of vitamin C and dietary fiber—three primary nutrients representing superfruit signatures and potential antioxidant qualities. Cherries also have an advantageously diverse profile of other micronutrients, giving them high value as a nutritious food. Calories are slightly higher in the sweet varieties due to the larger content of natural sugars (especially fructose and glucose), but the dense phenolic acids in the sour species, which create the tartness, may contribute additional phytochemical value in the diet. Of particular interest to medical scientists has been the anti-inflammatory properties shown to date in basic research on several cherry species.

Research Behind Cherries

The cherry's bright red color also advertises its high content of anthocyanin pigments such as cyanidin and peonidin glycosides. You can sometimes detect in the cherry taste a hint of cinnamon, which may derive from a polyphenol called cinnamic acid. Generally, sour cherries have higher concentrations of organic acids than sweet cherries, and some of these acids have antioxidant properties in test-tube experiments. This line of research has prompted specific investigations into how cherry polyphenols may affect inflammatory mechanisms seemingly involved at the onset of many diseases, including several types of cancer, diabetes, obesity, and metabolic syndrome.

FUN FACT!
The actual concentration of anthocyanins—the pigment polyphenol compounds giving cherries their beautiful red colors—varies among popular cultivars of cherries. Canadian government fruit researchers showed that the Sweetheart, Lapins, and Skeena cultivars had higher anthocyanin contents than Bing or Stoccata.

Cherries in the Research Pyramid

Because cherries are rich in anthocyanins, they are often linked with potential to treat diseases associated with inflammation, the onset mechanisms of which are thought to be particularly sensitive to anthocyanins. Accordingly, anthocyanin-rich fruit, including cherries as well as other berries such as the black raspberry and red grape, is a focus for inflammation research.

In early 2009, a phase II clinical trial sponsored by a company aptly named CherryPharm was launched to determine the effects of drinking cherry juice on pain perception in subjects with severe knee osteoarthritis. This human research was based on laboratory studies charting inflammation-induced pain behavior in rats. Results showed that tart cherry extracts reduce inflammation-induced pain and edema similarly to a dose of the pain-relief drug indomethacin. Although these studies indicate that tart cherry anthocyanins may have a beneficial role in the treatment of inflammatory pain, most of this research is based on test-tube or rat studies, meaning that progress remains within the lower half of the research pyramid.

Attaining clinical trial status means that a superfruit has reached the top of the pyramid, but, in early 2009, there is only one clinical trial active on cherry effects in humans. Thus, it is too early to conclude anything about antiarthritic pain prevention from cherry research.

Get Cherries into Your Diet!

Who doesn't like cherries as a whole fruit or as a taste? The fruit is just fun to eat fresh—and we don't have to wait for summer in the northern hemisphere anymore to do it. Now most people can get cherries year-round. Frozen, pitted ones are fine for nutrient content, but consuming them is not as delightful as eating the fruit fresh!

Eating ripe cherries is one of the true fruit pleasures of life and also provides a vitamin C boost. The long, firm stem—an eating convenience kindly supplied by Mother Nature, thank you—contributes a flair factor that makes cherries ideal as a garnish for practically any drink, smoothie, or dessert. Just a few cherries will give you a refreshing fruit break that is high in superfruit signatures and diverse nutrients. Kids love them, but urge care when disposing the large pits.

Whether for a whole-fruit cobbler made with whole grains, a garnish for your favorite cocktails or juices, or a side dish with salads, cherries rule in versatility and taste and are high in nutrient value, so let loose and use them more often in your regular diet! Six fresh cherries equal one fruit serving.

SOUR OR SWEET CHERRY SUPERFRUIT SCORE
Superfruit Score: 17/25
Rank Among 20 Superfruits: 9th (tied with papaya, blueberry, red raspberry, and seaberry)
Nutrient Content: 3/5
Phytochemical Content: 3/5
Medical Research Activity: 3/5
Position in Research Pyramid: 4/5
Popularity: 4/5

Red Raspberry (*Rubus idaeus*) NORTHWESTERN
UNITED STATES

Mother Nature wasn't joking around when she drew the blueprint for red raspberries. Delicate in both structure and taste, the red raspberry is a storehouse of nutrients packed in a unique, tasty, exotic form that distinguishes it among superfruits as a beautiful garnish for desserts and snacks.

Closely related to its superfruit cousins, the blackberry and black raspberry, red raspberry is a *Rubus* member of the rose family, *Rosaceae*. This group of fruits is characterized by its many individual drupelets, each like a small berry with one seed. The dozens of individual drupelets in one *Rubus* berry contribute extra skin, seeds, and pectin, which result in high dietary fiber and micronutrient value. This design places the red raspberry among the highest fiber-content plant foods known. The red raspberry is approximately 20 percent fiber by total weight!

WHY NOT BLACK RASPBERRIES?

Black raspberries are not included among the top twenty superfruits because they contain higher phenolic acid contents, are therefore sour if not bitter in taste, and are generally not enjoyed as much for fresh eating as the red species. Also, there is a limited supply of black raspberries in North America as this species has not been well crossbred to increase its resistance to plant diseases. Accordingly, farmers have not invested in black raspberries as a plant with higher disease risk and lower yield.

Why Red Raspberries Are Super

Red raspberries are one of the plant world's richest sources of vitamins C and K, the essential mineral manganese, and dietary fiber. Contents of vitamin A (from seed carotenoids), B vitamins 1 through 3 (thiamin, riboflavin, niacin, respectively), iron, calcium, and potassium are also at good levels.

Preliminary studies have shown evidence of red raspberry effects against intestinal pathogens and inflammatory mechanisms. These properties have been ascribed to the anthocyanin content, particularly the numerous cyanidin glycosides and ellagitannins, which are strongly linked to inhibiting mechanisms that initiate inflammation.

Red raspberries are good for more than just eating, though. Oil extracted from red raspberry seeds is popular as a skin moisturizer high in vitamins C and E, alpha-linolenic acid (omega-3 fatty acid), and linoleic acid (omega-6 fatty acid), with potent sun-blocking and healing properties.

Research Behind Red Raspberries

Red raspberries contain dense contents of ellagic acid, ellagitannins, and several other polyphenols under active research for potential health benefits as anti-inflammatory factors. These phenolic compounds have importance in research on diseases that start first with inflammation, such as cancer, chronic arthritis, Alzheimer's disease, diabetes, and obesity. In research done at Cornell University, scientists studying four cultivars of red raspberry identified differences in polyphenol content that were directly related to the color intensity of the respective juices. The color of the juice correlated well to the anthocyanin contents of each raspberry cultivar. In the same studies, proliferation of human liver cancer cells—as part of a laboratory test of potential anticancer activity—was significantly suppressed by the raspberry polyphenols.

Red Raspberries in the Research Pyramid

Both red and black raspberries are actively being investigated for phytochemicals that may hold benefits as future therapeutic agents. Certain antidisease properties have been isolated in experimental models.

Although there are no clinical studies to date proving these effects in humans, medical research shows that regularly consuming raspberries imparts a likely benefit against inflammation, pain, cancer onset mechanisms, cardiovascular disease, diabetes, allergies, age-related cognitive decline, and degeneration of eyesight with aging.

The research star is the *black* raspberry (either of two distinct, closely related species called *Rubus occidentalis* and *Rubus leucodermis*), which is at the forefront of clinical trials testing berries for anticancer activity. Oral, esophageal (throat), and colon cancer trials are in process by Dr. Gary Stoner and fellow scientists at Ohio State University. In rat studies reported early in 2009, Dr. Stoner's group announced that extracts from the black raspberry could alter the activity of as many as thirty-six genes of the esophagus (the smooth muscle tube for swallowing); twenty-four were switched to a higher state, called "upregulated," and twelve were "downregulated." Among the upregulated genes were those associated with cell structure, cell-to-cell signaling, metabolism, and—intriguingly —contraction capability of the esophageal smooth muscle cells.

Get Red Raspberries into Your Diet!

Nutritious red raspberries are ideal both as an addition to many types of recipes and as a healthy fresh snack by the handful. The often-mentioned blackcap—the black raspberry—is cultivated in the northwestern United States but not on the same commercial scale as the red raspberry. Because its products have fewer consumer applications, it does not have the same popular following for fresh uses, mainly on account of its higher astringency, somewhat bitter taste, and limited supply.

Red raspberries do not have to be fresh to be nutritious; quick-frozen and canned raspberries retain most of the nutrient qualities of fresh fruit. Consumers will sometimes see quick-frozen products labeled either "flash frozen" or "IQF" (immediately and individually quick frozen).

Raspberry leaves are also valuable, as they contain many of the fruit's nutrients as well. Red raspberry leaves are popular in tea blends, providing a complementary delicate flavor and source of tannins that add tartness and possible antioxidant value to the beverage. Just ten raspberries equal one fruit serving.

RED RASPBERRY SUPERFRUIT SCORE
Superfruit Score: 17/25
Rank Among 20 Superfruits: 9th (tied with papaya, blueberry, cherry, and seaberry)
Nutrient Content: 3/5
Phytochemical Content: 4/5
Medical Research Activity: 3/5
Position in Research Pyramid: 3/5
Popularity: 4/5

Seaberry ("sea buckthorn," *Hippophae rhamnoides*)
RUSSIA, CHINA, INDIA

SUPERFRUIT SNAPSHOT
Nutrient Content: high in prebiotic fiber, antioxidant A-C-E vitamins, dietary minerals, phytosterols, omega-3 and -6 fats (in pulp and edible seeds)
Phytochemical Content: high in carotenoids (beta-carotene), polyphenols (quercetin, kaempferol, rutin, isorhamnetin, myricetin)
Color Code: orange-yellow

Most people outside northern Europe, Russia, and parts of Asia likely have not heard of the golden seaberry, arguably one of the most nutrient-dense and diverse of all superfruits. On the downside, its musky, lemon-like taste combined with hefty amounts of pulp oil and organic acids makes for an unhappy marriage of flavor and aroma. At best, this is a superfruit with an acquired taste, and a well-designed consumer product is needed to improve its mass appeal.

Despite the fruit's not so "flavorable" taste, the seaberry should still be classified as a superfruit because of its extensive nutritional profile, potential value in consumer products, and unique lemonlike taste appreciated by millions in Europe and Asia. From Scandinavia east across Asia to Japan and south to India, seaberry juice, wine, cordial, tea, jam, and flavor for food and drinks are common and popular.

Considering its exceptional hardiness, tolerance of poor soils and a range of climates, and ability to succeed both in the wild and through cultivation, the seaberry is one of the most promising superfruits for supplying nutrient content to malnutrition regions.

FUN FACT!
The U.S. Department of Agriculture began using the name seaberry for the fruit around 2004, when consumer interest started growing on a wider scale. Most scientists still prefer using the name sea buckthorn, as reflected in most of the medical literature about this plant. *Sea* comes from the berry's ability to thrive in sandy soils and salty air near seas of its native lands in Asia and Europe; *buck* is a reference to a botanical family of more than one hundred buckthorn shrub and tree species; and *thorn* is for the long, sharp thorns all along the branches of the shrub—which make the seaberry difficult to harvest mechanically.

Why Seaberries Are Super

Seaberry's botanical family, *Elaeagnaceae*, is part of the order *Rosales*, as are other nutritious superfruits such as strawberries, blackberries, and raspberries, as well as cherries, black plums, almonds, and apples. Botanically, the seaberry is in good company as a nutrient source!

Seaberry micronutrients comprise an impressive list of essential vitamins and dietary minerals. Particularly rare is their high content of all three antioxidant vitamins—A (from the orange-yellow pigmented carotenoids, which are especially high in beta-carotene), C, and E (from the oil content in the pulp and seeds). The high concentration of the three antioxidant vitamins emphasizes the significant food value of seaberries, as these "ACE" vitamins have multiple roles in maintaining health—and you get the full high-dose trio in just one fruit— rare even among superfruits.

In addition, the essential dietary minerals calcium, iron, potassium, manganese, and magnesium are exceptionally high in content. Phytosterols and omega-3 fat sources (from alpha-linolenic acid) also are present in good levels. A negative dietary feature is the high amount of an undesired saturated fat, palmitic acid (about 30 percent of total fats), in seaberry fruit pulp. However, palmitic acid—mainly from the pulp oil compartment—has value for skin health, especially if applied externally as a lotion product. The fats from both the pulp and seeds are rich in omega-3, -6, and -9 fatty acids and dense in nutrient value, making them of further interest for product development by manufacturers of skin creams, lotions, soaps, balms, and hair-care products.

Research Behind Seaberries

The brilliant orange-yellow berry skins indicate a dense concentration of dietary carotenoids in seaberries, particularly beta-carotene, which converts to vitamin A in the body. Rich in a variety of organic acids, seaberries also have high phenolic contents, making this berry species exceptional among superfruits for having both major kinds of pigments in high concentration. As bioactive compounds best known as potential antioxidants, carotenoids and polyphenols are also thought to be involved in various organ and cellular processes. One 2009 study by Japanese scientists showed that seaberry pulp powder fed daily over two months to rats with severe cardiovascular disease could reduce the symptoms. This research points to a potential benefit from having seaberries in the diet for humans with cardiovascular disorders.

Perhaps because of such exceptional nutrient content, especially vitamin E and omega-3, -6, and -7 fatty acids, seaberry seed oils have been well studied in Finnish, Chinese, and Russian medical research. These studies address a variety of disease models: inflammation, skin injuries, vision disorders, cancer, thrombosis, and bacterial and fungal infections.

Seaberries in the Research Pyramid

Programs of human research in eastern Europe, China, and India have illustrated positive effects of seaberry therapeutic applications in limited clinical trials. Mainstream Western science, on the other hand, appears to be more skeptical, as the results are not typically cross-validated by studies in "first-world" clinical research countries acceptable to the FDA or EFSA, the regulatory bodies that screen applications for health claims and assure product safety for the public. For example, a diet containing seaberry and other fruits, herbs, honey, and grape seed extract was found by Romanian scientists to lower the risk of breast cancer in women, indicating that a diet enriched with seaberry bioactive compounds might complement treatment of cancer patients. Although promising, this interesting research has not been confirmed.

Get Seaberries into Your Diet!

If you happen to be in northern Europe, India, or Southeast Asia, you probably can find seaberry products in the general consumer market. However, these products are only available in North America through specialty health stores and Internet sites, but distribution is expanding year by year. Take note that one has to be completely open when trying to eat or drink a seaberry preparation. I take a favorable view toward seaberry products, but I still have difficulty with the raw berries or juice! Seaberry flavors are just too oily, musky, and lemonlike for most palates.

This hitch does not mean that the fruit has no potential as a superfruit product. Asians, Indians, and Europeans enjoy seaberry in various formats—juice, nutrition bars, tea, oil capsules—and it does add a flavor edge to blended beverages and fruit products such as sauces and marmalades. Making these offerings more nutritious with a lemony taste is perhaps where seaberry will gain its place eventually in world markets. Just four to eight ounces of juice is approximately one fruit serving.

SEABERRY SUPERFRUIT SCORE
Superfruit Score: 17/25
Rank Among 20 Superfruits: 9th (tied with papaya, blueberry, cherry, and red raspberry)
Nutrient Content: 5/5
Phytochemical Content: 5/5
Medical Research Activity: 3/5
Position in Research Pyramid: 2/5
Popularity: 2/5

Guava, green and red ("strawberry" guava)
(*PSIDIUM GUAJAVA* AND *PSIDIUM LITTORALE* VAR. *CATTLEIANUM*) CENTRAL AND SOUTH AMERICA

SUPERFRUIT SNAPSHOT
Nutrient Content: high in prebiotic fiber, antioxidant A-C-E vitamins, dietary minerals
Phytochemical Content: high in carotenoids (beta-cryptoxanthin, beta-carotene, lycopene), polyphenols (anthocyanins)
Color Code: red, green

Although there are about one hundred species of guava, and it is popular in many tropical regions, this superfruit is not often seen on the produce stands of major grocery chains in the United States or Canada. One way of getting to know its use for your diet is to try juices, jams, fruit leathers, or sauces that can be found on the Internet. Its limited North American distribution might have something to do with lack of access to the most favored species and problems of fruit flies being attracted to the appealing guava fragrance. Some species of guava may have a coarse skin and a bitter, almost rindlike flavor, while others may be soft and sweet. Across species, the skin can be any color, with yellow or maroon fruits usually preferred over green (may indicate unripe fruit). Guava pulp may be sweet and white or strawberry-like in appearance, with the red indicating the phytochemical presence of the carotenoid lycopene.

Why Guavas Are Super

Guavas are often ranked among the most valued superfruits, being rich in signature nutrients, especially vitamin C and prebiotic fiber but also vitamins A, E, and K, as well as omega-3 and -6 polyunsaturated fatty acids (mainly in the seeds, which must be blended or chewed to allow for ingestion of the omega fats). A single serving of green guava offers exceptional vitamin C content, about 200 mg, which is twice the daily value—more vitamin C than the flavorful strawberry guava. Both species have good levels of several dietary minerals and a favorable, low-calorie nutrient profile. Guavas are dense in content of pectin, a valued prebiotic fiber. Red species of guava have high carotenoid content, particularly beta-cryptoxanthin, which converts to vitamin A in the body, and lycopene, a candidate antioxidant.

Research Behind Guavas

Guavas contain both major classes of antioxidant pigments, carotenoids and polyphenols—the latter occurring in more density as lycopene in fruits with red-orange flesh. Because of this significant dietary value, they are of interest in medical research on possible antioxidant or other cell effects controlled by carotenoids and polyphenols providing pro-vitamin A value. Guava is a regionally important food for a range of practical applications due to its high nutrient levels, such as for beverages, meal garnishes, desserts, and snacks.

Guava leaves in particular have been a subject for preliminary research to identify potential antidisease properties. Extracts from leaves or bark are implicated in controlling mechanisms of cancer, bacterial infections, and inflammation. Essential oils from guava leaves have also shown anticancer activity in laboratory experiments.

Guavas in the Research Pyramid

The high content of lycopene in most red species of guava attracts the attention of researchers investigating the potential health values of this candidate carotenoid antioxidant. Lycopene's chemical structure includes numerous double bonds, which are known from test-tube science to make this substance highly reactive toward oxygen radicals, and this antioxidant activity probably contributes to the promise for lycopene as an anticancer agent. As a rich lycopene source, guava is a leading dietary candidate for combating cancer.

Known better in traditional medical practices than in conventional research, guava has been associated particularly with broad antimicrobial and antiviral properties and is still under study in the laboratory to confirm these therapeutic effects. Mexican scientists showed that guava extracts and metabolites from leaves and fruit have useful pharmacological applications, including treatment of intestinal disorders, allergies, inflammation, and pain, supporting its common traditional uses. This research, however, has not been confirmed in subsequent studies by Western scientists, thus relegating guava to the lower two steps in the health claims research pyramid.

Get Guavas into Your Diet!

Guava has an attention-grabbing sweet citruslike fragrance, giving it purchase as a high-nutrient dessert. Because of the fruit's significant polysaccharide content, boiled guava yields gels useful for making candies, preserves, jellies, jams, marmalades, juices, and frescas—a refreshing blend of fruit juice with carbonated soda. Guava juice is particularly popular in Mexico, the Middle East, and South Africa and is now often seen in Canadian and American grocery stores. Guava sauces and salsas are popular in Central American and Caribbean countries. Just half a guava equals one serving.

GUAVA SUPERFRUIT SCORE
Superfruit Score: 16/25
Rank Among 20 Superfruits: 14th
Nutrient Content: 5/5
Phytochemical Content: 4/5
Medical Research Activity: 2/5
Position in Research Pyramid: 2/5
Popularity: 3/5

Blackberry (*Rubus ursinus*) WORLDWIDE IN NORTHERN TEMPERATE ZONES, MEXICO

The blackberry is a member of the *Rubus* family of berries, which also includes red and black raspberries. It is one of nature's more interesting fruits and is actually not a berry but rather an "aggregate fruit" comprising many small fruits in lobules called drupelets, each containing a seed enriched with nutrients and omega-3 fats (about 20 percent of seed fat content).

An aggressively growing vine sometimes called a cane, the blackberry plant may be one of the world's most prolific growers, as this perennial spreads rapidly via ground trailers and long, arching canes producing abundant fruit in late summer.

Why Blackberries Are Super

Blackberry signature nutrients stand out as particularly enriched: vitamin C, dietary fiber, manganese, and vitamin K are all at about 20 percent of daily value per serving and are combined with a broad profile of other nutrients in good content. A hidden quality not enjoyed by everyone is the presence of nutrient-laden seeds throughout each berry. If you don't mind the crunchy surprise in each bite, make sure to chew these seeds well to gain the maximum yield of their nutrient contents.

Research Behind Blackberries

Blackberries are considered enriched in antioxidants, particularly for their significant amounts of polyphenols—ellagitannins, cyanidins, and other anthocyanins. Presumably, these compounds account for the relatively high value for antioxidant capacity shown by test-tube studies.

Although research on blackberries has been limited, increasing attention is being directed to the potential anticancer effect of their anthocyanins—particularly cyanidins from the pulp and ellagitannins from seeds. In a 2008 report from the University of British Columbia, blackberry anthocyanins, among which 80 percent are cyanidin glycosides, were effective at inhibiting onset mechanisms of colon cancer cells in culture. Similar studies by Italian scientists showed that blackberry cyanidins were protective against damage by peroxynitrite radicals in human umbilical blood vessels, a laboratory model for vascular injury.

A study published in 2006 in the *American Journal of Clinical Nutrition* by scientists at the University of Oslo, Norway, showed blackberry at the very top of more than one thousand antioxidant foods consumed in the United States. Although this rank is disputed by some scientists, blackberries are regarded as among the most antioxidant-enriched fruits.

Blackberries in the Research Pyramid

As with many other dark berries, the blackberry's contents of phenolic acids, especially pigment anthocyanins—which give the blackberry among the darkest colors existing in the plant world—lead the medical research on antidisease mechanisms. Anthocyanins are linked with anti-inflammatory effects that may be at the origin of numerous unrelated diseases, such as diabetes, cancer, and Alzheimer's disease. In an alternate direction, Mexican scientists have developed a use for blackberries in medical imaging procedures: the berries are so deeply pigmented by anthocyanins that they were implemented as an oral contrast agent for magnetic resonance imaging to assess gastric and digestive functions.

Despite their being in the medical literature for nearly seventy years, blackberries have not been intensely studied for their potential health benefits in humans until recently. In recognition of their exceptional cyanidin pigmentation (accounting for their near-black color), blackberries and other *Rubus* species are now a major focus of research on anthocyanins for inhibiting mechanisms of inflammation, cancer, and cardiovascular diseases. Thanks to the blackberry's avid growth capabilities, supplies of the fruit are abundant, assuring ample research material for future studies.

Get Blackberries into Your Diet!

Blackberries are almost always eaten raw. Dried fruits are not practical, and juices have not been widely popularized, although blackberry wine has a devoted following. The taste can be mellow, delicious, and almost irresistible, but the presence of seeds discourages some people who do not like coming across the firm, chewy kernels in virtually every drupelet. These unavoidable seeds are nutrient-laden features, however, so count them as part of the fruit experience, and enjoy them—just make sure you crunch and grind them to assure optimal extraction of the nutrients.

In many parts of the world during late summer, wild-growing blackberries offer the general public a cost-free, delicious source of fresh fruit brimming with promising anthocyanins and nutrients. Just eight fresh blackberries equal one fruit serving.

BLACKBERRY SUPERFRUIT SCORE
Superfruit Score: 15/25
Rank Among 20 Superfruits: 15th
Nutrient Content: 4/5
Phytochemical Content: 4/5
Medical Research Activity: 3/5
Position in Research Pyramid: 1/5
Popularity: 3/5

Blackcurrant (*Ribes nigrum*) NORTHERN EUROPE AND UNITED KINGDOM, NEW ZEALAND, CANADIAN PRAIRIES

SUPERFRUIT SNAPSHOT

Nutrient Content: high in prebiotic fiber, antioxidant vitamins C and E (in edible seeds), dietary minerals

Phytochemical Content: high in polyphenols (anthocyanins—particularly delphinidin and cyanidin glycosides and rutinosides, quercetin, hydroxycinnamic acid, proanthocyanidins)

Color Code: black-purple

Long popular in Europe, the blackcurrant is one superfruit that has a sharp, distinctive flavor—often preferred in baking hot cross buns during the Easter season in many Western countries. It is a primary ingredient in the beverage Ribena—which many consider one of the richest-tasting fruit juices known—as well as in popular beverage mixes used in Britain and mainland Europe for cider, Guinness beer, and a western European soft drink called cassis, made from blackcurrant juice.

Why Blackcurrants Are Super

Blackcurrants have extraordinarily high vitamin C content (302 percent of daily value per 100 g); good DV levels of dietary fiber, potassium, phosphorus, iron, and vitamin B_5; and a broad range of other essential nutrients. Blackcurrant seeds are also rich in many nutrients, and seed oils have value in nutraceuticals and cosmetics.

Blackcurrants have regional importance across the world, with Scandinavian countries, Poland, New Zealand, and Scotland devoting special efforts to research and crop development. In Britain, there is a Blackcurrant Foundation devoted to promoting the fruit as the world's number one superfruit. For more information, visit blackcurrantfoundation.co.uk.

Research Behind Blackcurrants

Polyphenols in blackcurrant fruit, mainly anthocyanins, have been shown experimentally to inhibit inflammation mechanisms under study for the origin of several diseases, including cancer, chronic arthritis, and diabetes. Similarly, studies using an enriched fraction of simple sugars from blackcurrants, such as arabinose and galactose, fed to mice with cancer demonstrated slower growth of the tumors.

Because currants are unusually rich in anthocyanins, scientists have endeavored to determine when the anthocyanin content peaks during maturation of the fruit while still on the bush. The highest amounts of anthocyanins were found in overripe blackcurrants of breeds called Vakariai and Ben Alder.

Blackcurrants in the Research Pyramid

Blackcurrants are being studied in laboratory experiments to test for potential activity against heart disease, cancer, microbial infections, and neurological disorders such as Alzheimer's disease. In a 2008 study in Italy, blackcurrants were used in a nutraceutical product called Pantescal to study subjects allergic to common airborne allergens, revealing that allergy biomarkers were decreased by the treatment.

Despite research interest in blackcurrants dating back to 1917, the number of publications has been limited, totaling only 190 over nearly a century, indicating that progress up the research pyramid is not at a significant pace. Nevertheless, blackcurrants offer three major superfruit signatures in very high content—vitamin C, dietary fiber, and polyphenols—and so will continue to attract research interest and eventually climb higher in research accomplishment.

Get Blackcurrants into Your Diet!

Having been deemed a possible vector of pine tree disease, blackcurrants were once banned from cultivation in the United States (and still are by some states), but blackcurrant farming is making a comeback in America and the prairies of western Canada. The growing supply is now providing many supermarkets with dried bulk-bin fruit ideal for snacking and use in a variety of recipes. You can also find blackcurrant juice as part of blends with grape, cranberry, or pomegranate juice, as well as jams and syrups.

Dried blackcurrants are comparable in taste to Thompson raisins, though they are less sweet and smaller. They occasionally have noticeable seeds (which I consider a bonus, as seeds harbor valuable nutrient contents!). The fresh fruit and juice, however, often are regarded by consumers as having an almost bitter taste. Still, my mother loved to put lots of blackcurrants in her famous hot cross buns and pies, which were always a family favorite. One serving equals about sixty dried blackcurrants or a four-ounce glass of juice.

BLACKCURRANT SUPERFRUIT SCORE
Superfruit Score: 14/25
Rank Among 20 Superfruits: 16th (tied with date)
Nutrient Content: 4/5
Phytochemical Content: 3/5
Medical Research Activity: 2/5
Position in Research Pyramid: 2/5
Popularity: 3/5

Date (*Phoenix dactylifera*) NORTHERN AFRICA, MIDDLE EAST

SUPERFRUIT SNAPSHOT

Nutrient Content: high in prebiotic fiber, vitamin B6 (pyridoxine), several dietary minerals, phytosterols

Phytochemical Content: high in carotenoids (beta-carotene), polyphenols (anthocyanins, oligomeric proanthocyanidins, tannins, luteolin, quercetin, apigenin)

Color Code: tan-red, orange-yellow

Recognizable from the palm trees of desert oases, dates have been a staple of the Middle Eastern diet over recorded history. Now cultivated especially in Morocco, Saudi Arabia, and Egypt, they are burgeoning in popularity in Western countries as a convenient dried fruit for garnishes and snacks, making them an appetizing and high-nutrient, but high-calorie, superfruit.

Almost a perfectly sized "finger food" in about the shape of a thumb, dates come in a large variety of cultivars, moisture and sugar content, and colors from tans to dark browns to near red or orange-brown.

Dates are popular for use in pastries and other baked goods, smoothies, sandwich spreads, party snacks, salads, and appetizers. Macerated date chunks are often used for cooking, as are date paste and flour. Add to that roster sweets and snacks (such as date nut roll), chocolate-coated and stuffed dates (with crushed nuts), date jams, date butter and cream, and date preserves. Further, with the pit removed, a date becomes a perfect little container for making fun food for the kids: peanut butter, marmalade, fruit jams, or honey stuff neatly into the pit cavity!

Why Dates Are Super

Date pulp is low in fat and protein but rich in sugars, mainly fructose and glucose, making it a potent source of caloric energy. It contains excellent amounts of amino acids for protein; dietary minerals such as selenium, potassium, calcium, magnesium, manganese, and iron; several B vitamins; vitamin C; omega fatty acids; phytosterols; and both insoluble and prebiotic fiber. Among the best-known varieties of dates are the Deglet Noor and Medjool—I prefer the Deglet Noor. Nutritiondata.com, a great resource for nutrient contents of many foods, rates Deglet Noor dates as a high-nutrient source, whereas the often pricey Medjool dates, perhaps more popular due to their sweetness, are substantially lower in nutrient content and higher in calories. Numerous other varieties are entering Western markets.

Because dates are easy to grow, transport, and store, and have excellent nutrient value, they have become one of the primary focus foods for development and donation in humanitarian relief from more prosperous countries such as Saudi Arabia to the world's poorest, malnourished nations. Such programs are sponsored by the World Health Organization, the World Food and Agriculture Organization, the World Labor Organization, the World Food Program, UNICEF, UNESCO, and the U.N. Development Program.

FUN FACT!
If you've encountered date pits, you know their usual fate—they are promptly discarded. But wait: a nutritional study of date pits has documented their exceptional nutrient density, especially of protein, dietary fiber, and omega oils composed mainly of oleic acid, the same omega-9 monounsaturated fat famous in olive oil. Date pits may offer an inexpensive nutrient and oil source from what is currently a waste material. Simply through extraction or pulp processing of the pits, some future entrepreneur will recover those inedible pits and transform them into useful food products!

Research Behind Dates

Both carotenoids and polyphenols have been identified in dates. This rare combination of compounds may contribute antioxidant and other properties that could lower disease risk. Otherwise, the focus of research on dates has been their value as a nutrient-rich food staple and malnutrition rescue food. The date palm is one of the most prolific and least costly producers of food per hectare, with worldwide cultivation exceeding three million tons.

The date fruit consists of 70 percent carbohydrates (mostly sugars), making it one of the most calorie-rich, high-nutrient fruits available. With the present uncertainty in the world food supply and the expected increase in demand from food production countries, the date could be a premium source of high nutritional and caloric value, and it preserves easily for shipping and storage.

Dates provide more than *3,000 calories per kilogram*! Look at these striking comparisons with other fruits and foods in calories per kilogram: apricot, 520; banana, 970; orange, 480; cooked rice, 1,800; wheat bread, 2,295; beef (without fat), 2,245. This tilt of the balance indicates that further horticultural research to expand production of date cultivars with high nutritional value will be important for the future food supply. Researchers with the Department of Health and Human Sciences at London Metropolitan University, in the United Kingdom, have weighed in with a published paper entitled "The Fruit of the Date Palm: Its Possible Use as the Best Food for the Future?"

Dates in the Research Pyramid

Dates have been undeveloped in health research, possibly because the countries of Africa and the Middle East in which they are staples of the diet are not significantly involved in global medical research. Other than the generally appreciated nutrient value, few health-related implications have been established, although the fruit would certainly be valuable for alleviating malnutrition in impoverished countries. One recent study by scientists in Abu Dhabi indicated that date pit extracts had strong ability to inhibit the infection rate of *Pseudomonas* phage bacteria, a diversified pathogen, and completely prevented bacterial breakage of cell membranes. Such research underscores the potential for using date pit extracts as antibacterial agents against human pathogens.

Get Dates into Your Diet!

It's the sweetness and pleasant chewiness that keeps me coming back to fill my shopping bag with dates. Fortunately, cultivars such as Deglet Noor are also among the most cost-effective dried fruit you can find! Plain and simple, they are an enjoyable eating experience, often made better by a topping of vanilla yogurt or as a snack with mixed nuts and fresh fruits. Be inventive: you can use date chunks in almost any salad, stir-fry, casserole, or dessert. As a dried—although somewhat sticky—fruit, they can be popped into a ziplock sandwich bag to carry along as a snack when you're on the move. Just four dates equal one fruit serving.

DATE SUPERFRUIT SCORE
Superfruit Score: 14/25
Rank Among 20 Superfruits: 16th (tied with blackcurrant)
Nutrient Content: 5/5
Phytochemical Content: 3/5
Medical Research Activity: 1/5
Position in Research Pyramid: 0/5
Popularity: 5/5

Pomegranate (*Punica granatum*) MEDITERRANEAN REGION, CALIFORNIA

SUPERFRUIT SNAPSHOT
Nutrient Content: high in dietary minerals, moderate vitamin C
Phytochemical Content: high in polyphenols called punicalagins (ellagitannins) and anthocyanins (red pigments)
Color Code: red

If it were not for the impressive progress that pomegranate juice is making along the health claims research pyramid, I might not have chosen the pomegranate for inclusion among superfruits. The intact fruit, which is about the size of a grapefruit, has a thick, hard, reddish outer rind and about six hundred seeds deep inside the internal white pith—the whole object of eating this superfruit is to get to the seeds. The seeds and surrounding juice-filled pulp, usually a deep red, are called arils in botany and are the juicy, edible prize for all your work in getting to them.

Think of an aril the way Mother Nature made it: it is a protective layer of water, trace nutrients, and defensive phytochemicals called punicalagins (a group of ellagitannin compounds thought to be strong antioxidants) contained in a barely noticeable sheath covering the seed.

FUN FACT!

To retrieve pomegranate arils, score around the fruit rind, pry the halves apart, and scoop out the red seeds, removing any of the light-colored pith. The arils tend to squirt when they pop, and you will invariably spray randomly while dissecting a pomegranate. A good way to avoid the squirting juices is to do the seed retrievals with the fruit completely submerged in a basin of water. The extracted seeds sink to the bottom, while the pith will mostly float and can be easily removed. After picking away the pith, pour the basin contents through a colander, and rinse with tap water to collect the arils. Then you're ready to store them refrigerated in a covered bowl for any use, even just as they are for a tasty, exotic snack and garnish. Given the antioxidant qualities of the aril juice, the refrigerated seeds preserve well over a long duration of storage.

Why Pomegranates Are Super

Pomegranate aril juice has only traces of nutrients, with vitamin C and potassium at moderate levels but nothing else of much nutritional content. The seed is where the nutrient prize lives. If chewed, the seeds deliver high levels of micronutrients, phytosterols, omega fatty acids, and fiber.

Regardless, the reputation of pomegranate as a superfruit is based entirely on its juice and polyphenol extract products, which are typically low in nutrient content, so it's always wise to check the Nutrition Facts panel on your favorite juice brand if nutrients are your goal.

The real surprise of pomegranate juice is the significant bioactivity shown in laboratory studies and in early-stage human clinical trials. This finding implies that pomegranate polyphenols, likely the ellagitannin molecules called punicalagins, are primed to be at the center of research interest for antidisease activity, a scientific field still evolving.

Research Behind Pomegranates

The simplicity of botanical design of the pomegranate aril focuses attention on its punicalagins unique to the aril juice. Punicalagins are bioactive in test-tube studies, showing potent antioxidant and anti-inflammatory properties. Pomegranate juice has the highest concentration of ellagitannins of any commonly consumed fruit juice. During digestion, ellagitannins are not absorbed intact into the blood but rather are broken down to ellagic acid, a powerful in vitro antioxidant under study for how it may affect human health.

Test-tube or animal studies of pomegranate juice or its ellagitannin extracts have shown significant activity in the following areas of disease investigation:

▶ Inflammation
▶ Cancer models, specifically in the prostate gland
▶ Growth of blood vessels in tumors
▶ Shear stress of vascular endothelial cells, a model for studying vascular disease
▶ Ultraviolet light–induced oxygen radicals in skin cells
▶ Several strains of bacteria
▶ A malarial parasite, *Plasmodium falciparum*

Pomegranate juice has also been shown in animal experiments to reduce high blood pressure, inhibit viral infections, and have antibacterial effects against dental plaque.

Pomegranates in the Research Pyramid

While medical research on pomegranates has existed for about sixty years, during which time more than three hundred research reports appeared, some 90 percent of these studies were published just in the last fifteen years, when global interest in pomegranate juice spiked.

The pomegranate has a vast history of traditional uses for all of its anatomical compartments—seed, juice, rind, leaf, flower, bark, and roots. Each has interesting extracts with biological activity. The juice, rind, and seed oil have demonstrated anti-inflammatory activity in laboratory experiments, including interference with tumor cell proliferation, invasion, and blood vessel growth.

Commercial pomegranate juice is being examined in numerous clinical trials to determine its potential use in controlling prostate gland hypertrophy, cancer, diabetes, the common cold, rhinoviral infections, and development of vascular disease. This is an achievement made possible almost exclusively by the dedication of manufacturers to have their juice products tested in clinical trials by independent scientists.

In preliminary human studies, use of pomegranate juice led to a decrease in levels of prostate-specific immune response after primary treatment with surgery or radiation, indicating that the juice may be beneficial as a stabilizing or preventive agent against prostate cancer.

Use of pomegranate juice or extracts in prostate cancer studies has become the main focus of current clinical trials being conducted at numerous cancer centers in the United States, such as the M. D. Anderson Cancer Center, in Houston; the University of California, Los Angeles; and Washington University, in St. Louis.

Get Pomegranates into Your Diet!

Once the arils are out of the fruit and in your mouth, most people would agree they are quite enjoyable. They also are versatile and exotic for garnishing dishes; when you're entertaining, the bold red spheres are a hallmark that you have served your guests something special. Pomegranate seed arils add sparkle to appetizers, beverage garnishes, salads, main-dish vegetables, and desserts.

Fortunately, numerous manufacturers simplify getting the prized aril juice into the convenience of bottles, although usually at a price relatively high compared with grape, orange, or tomato juice, which offer superior nutritional value. Pomegranate juice often is included in a blend with Concord grape, blueberry, or cranberry juice. A little like red raspberry juice (and with similar phytochemicals), the taste of pomegranate juice and its storied history are what drive sales of this exotic superfruit juice. About eight ounces of 100 percent pomegranate juice equals one fruit serving.

POMEGRANATE SUPERFRUIT SCORE
Superfruit Score: 13/25
Rank Among 20 Superfruits: 18th (tied with açaí)
Nutrient Content: 1/5
Phytochemical Content: 2/5
Medical Research Activity: 3/5
Position in Research Pyramid: 4/5
Popularity: 3/5

Açaí (*Euterpe oleracea* Mart.) BRAZIL

SUPERFRUIT SNAPSHOT
Nutrient Content: high in protein, prebiotic fiber, antioxidant vitamin E, dietary minerals, phytosterols, omega fats, lignans; high in palmitic acid, a saturated fat (negative feature)
Phytochemical Content: high in polyphenols (numerous anthocyanins, especially cyanidin glycosides, proanthocyanidins)
Color Code: dark purple

Açaí (pronounced: ah-sigh-EE) is a dark blue-purple berry that grows in dense clusters at the apex of açaí palm trees in equatorial rainforests of Brazil and Panama. Available in the United States only since the late 1990s, it became popular as a powder additive for smoothies and then later, when sweetened or blended with other fruit juices, gained recognition as a juice, sometimes likened to an alluring cross in flavor between blueberries and chocolate.

The freeze-dried powder, expensive for most consumers at about $27 per pound, is nevertheless popular for manufacturing uses in smoothies, granola bars, cereals, and chocolate and as a flavor-color additive for beverages. Some American processors retain the pasteurized berry pulp as a frozen puree, which is useful in manufacturing sorbet, ice cream, gelato, jam, and yogurt products. Juice and oils are extracted from the puree raw material for manufacturing needs.

A barrage of media hype occurred when açaí was announced on Oprah's show in 2004 as the world's number one superfood. Maybe when it's fresh off the palm tree—the way indigenous Amazonians have used it for centuries—it is right up there among top superfruits for overall nutrient density and food value.

But açaí has three important detractions for harvesting and processing: first, only about 20 percent of each berry is edible due to the exceptionally large single seed which, itself, is inedible; second, açaí requires special post-harvest handling in the humid heat of equatorial Brazil; and third, açaí anthocyanins—the pigments giving its distinct dark purple color—readily degrade into brown pigmentation, making retention of the popular purple color a critical manufacturing challenge.

For safety, economical storage and shipping, açaí must be quickly irradiated or pasteurized after removal from the tree, then processed into either a powder (by the expensive method of freeze-drying) or a frozen pulp puree. Irradiation and/or pasteurization are required safety procedures to destroy microbes, but also diminish vitamins and other nutrients, which become further reduced by subsequent steps in processing. The reduction of natural açaí nutrients is evident from the Nutrition Facts panel on many commercial juice products—in most cases showing few if any nutrients.

Because of the special handling required for this fruit, its naturally low pulp volume and high saturated fat (23 percent palmitic acid) content, degradation of the anthocyanin pigments, and unpalatable flavor of the raw fruit, you may never see fresh or whole frozen açaí berries in an American supermarket, a constraint on its appeal as a superfruit available as a whole food to the public. Also, exportation of seeds or cuttings that would permit propagation and horticultural enhancement of açaí palms in other countries is currently restricted by the Brazilian government (presumably, to preserve Brazil's reputation as "home" of the açaí). It's possible that frozen pulp of açaí will become more available as an imported retail product that best retains the exceptional nutrient value of the raw, fresh fruit.

Why Açaí Berries Are Super

When fresh or as a freeze-dried powder processed soon after harvesting, açaí bears an exceptional nutrient profile, being particularly dense in protein, dietary fiber (highest fiber content among plant foods described to date), vitamin E, and beta-sitosterol, a phytosterol with cholesterol-lowering properties. Mainly because of the exceptional fat levels, açaí is a significant calorie source.

The research excitement about açaí has derived from its prodigious content of polyphenols—anthocyanins, proanthocyanidins, and tannins. These polyphenols collectively create strong antioxidant effects in test-tube studies.

NOT ALL TESTS ARE EQUAL

In a test-tube method called ORAC (oxygen radical absorbance capacity), freeze-dried açaí powder scored the highest ORAC level yet determined among fruits, a result that incited a storm of marketing literature declaring that açaí products have the highest antioxidant health value of any food. The bad news is that there are limitations to that ORAC value as we know it (see Appendix A). Antioxidant properties determined in test tubes are unlikely to have the same antioxidant roles in the human body. Further, the comparisons of açaí ORAC with other fruits are not valid since the fruit preparations were not identical across all tests.

As a nutrient-dense, polyphenol-enriched fruit, açaí is certain to be manufactured in future nutritious food and beverage products. Just as certain, more research is still needed to understand optimal processing methods for preserving its potential health properties.

Research Behind Açaí Berries

Açaí's rich blue-purple color advertises its high content of anthocyanins, a class of plant polyphenols under study as potential anti-disease agents. Five chemically different anthocyanins, particularly cyanidins, and at least a dozen other polyphenols have been isolated, including a high content of proanthocyanidins linked to possible anti-disease effects, such as in bacterial infections, onset of cancer, and inflammation.

In test-tube studies on açaí anthocyanins and other polyphenols, Dr. Steve Talcott showed that growth of leukemia cells was inhibited, indicating a similar effect from anthocyanins on cancer cells as can be seen with red and black raspberries, cranberries, and blueberries. His subsequent research at Texas A&M University proved that colon cancer cells were inhibited by açaí polyphenols in vitro, giving promise that açaí may eventually prove useful as a dietary agent for lowering risk of various types of cancer in humans.

Numerous members of the polyphenol family have been identified in açaí, but their roles as anti-disease agents or dietary nutrients remain insufficiently evaluated. Particularly in the harvested fruit, these anthocyanins tend to polymerize (individual anthocyanins join in chains of dozens to hundreds), causing the fruit pigmentation to change from purple to an unattractive brown. Research is continuing in laboratory models to study the effects of pure, native anthocyanins on cancer and cardiovascular disease experimental models.

Açaí Berries in the Research Pyramid

Although Brazilian research interest in açaí has existed sparsely over decades, it was only in 2004 that the first research papers were published in American journals, igniting Western research interest on a wider scale. By comparison with other superfruits, açaí is the least understood of all and is only in the most preliminary stages of investigation.

As basic research on açaí has such a short history, this fruit has not been tested under a variety of experimental conditions and, accordingly, does not yet have scientific substantiation comparable to better-validated superfruits. However, açaí's combination of diverse phytochemical content with exceptional nutrient composition guarantees this fruit a place in future research and product development.

Get Açaí Berries into Your Diet!

By itself as a powder or in 100 percent juice form, açaí berries are low in natural sugars, very tart, and unpleasant for taste, most probably as a result of the dense phenolic acids and minimal sugars. Commercially blended or sweetened açaí juices have become popular due to their rich, blueberry-like appearance and taste. The products you will find for sale contain some sweetening agent or other fruits and their sugars to offset the natural acidity. Also, to satisfy stringent aesthetics needed for bottled fruit juices, the valued monounsaturated oil (oleic fatty acid, also found in olive oil), vitamin E, and dietary fiber of the açaí berries must be removed in clear açaí juice, making such products considerably less nutritious than the fruit promises. This conclusion indicates the smoothie using freeze-dried whole powder containing these nutrients is probably the optimal nutritional format available to the general consumer.

AÇAÍ SUPERFRUIT SCORE
Superfruit Score: 13/25
Rank Among 20 Superfruits: 18th (tied with pomegranate)
Nutrient Content: 5/5
Phytochemical Content: 4/5
Medical Research Activity: 1/5
Position in Research Pyramid: 0/5 (Western medical research began in 2004)
Popularity: 3/5

Dried plum (prune, *Prunus domesticus*) CALIFORNIA, MEDITERRANEAN BASIN

SUPERFRUIT SNAPSHOT
Nutrient Content: high in protein, prebiotic and insoluble fiber, lignans, antioxidant vitamins A and C, dietary minerals, phytosterols
Phytochemical Content: high in total carotenoids and polyphenols (anthocyanins, catechins, proanthocyanidins, chlorogenic acid)
Color Code: black-purple

Dried plums deserve more respect than they get. Their convenience for snacks or meal garnishes, combined with their richness in vitamins A (from carotenoids), B, and K and prebiotic fiber, brings them into the league of superfruits. Dried plums are not any more nutritious than the fresh black plums you can often find on the produce shelf—just more convenient, versatile, and loved over generations!

Worldwide, more than a thousand cultivated varieties of plums are pitted and dried to make prunes, which are usually eaten as a single-fruit snack. Prune juice and puree are also versatile as consumer and industrial products. Prunes are frequently used in cooking for both sweet and savory dishes, as well as with yogurt. Stewed or in a hot compote, prunes are favored as a dessert. They have a wide variety of uses in traditional meals, snacks, and side dishes.

FUN FACT!
The highest prune production occurs in the Californian Sacramento and San Joaquin valleys, which together produce more prunes than the rest of the world combined. Nearly all the U.S. supply and 60 percent of the world's supply come from California.

Why Dried Plums Are Super

A dried fruit outstanding to just be enjoyed for its soft texture, chewing, and rich taste, the prune has excellent micronutrient diversity. It's rich in both prebiotic (soluble viscous) and insoluble dietary fiber (including lignans), protein, vitamins, and several essential minerals. Prunes are notable for having a low glycemic load and so are recommended for suppressing appetite.

Research on prunes or their polyphenol extracts has documented the ability to inhibit inflammatory mechanisms and cancer cell proliferation. As with other superfruits, this type of polyphenol research emphasizes the potential of using these fruits as dietary aids for lowering disease risk.

Research Behind Dried Plums

The laxative action for which prunes and prune juice are well known could be explained by the high content of sorbitol, a sugar alcohol that stimulates water influx to the intestinal tract to slow digestion, giving prunes a low glycemic impact. Prunes contain carotenoids and boast significant polyphenol content, mainly as anthocyanins, proanthocya-nidins, and neochlorogenic acid, which are under study for a variety of biological functions, such as anti-inflammatory activity, pain treatment, and potential anticancer activity. Dietary studies with prunes in mice and rats showed specific effects on peripheral vascular disease, osteopo-rosis, and colon cancer.

Overall, the research effort to identify health properties of the dried plum relies on two primary signatures for superfruit status—dietary fiber and mixed polyphenols. A Japanese research group has done much of the work on polyphenols, establishing a list of candidates for antioxidant or other cellular effects of prune compounds. Oligomeric proanthocyani-dins, chlorogenic acid, caffeoylquinic acid, various other phenolic acids, and lignans have exhibited antioxidant activity in test-tube studies. Each of these compounds is under research for potential beneficial roles sup-porting human health.

Dried Plums in the Research Pyramid

In laboratory experiments, prune extracts inhibit cholesterol synthesis and oxidation of lipids and thus might serve to lower the risk of chronic vascular diseases. A limited study by nutritionists at the University of California, Davis, examining men with high blood cholesterol provided evidence for this effect, showing that eating twelve prunes a day for eight weeks reduced overall blood cholesterol levels.

The high fiber value, polyphenols, and good content of dietary min-erals in prunes is a combination that has promise for reducing risk of chronic inflammation, osteoporosis, cardiovascular diseases, and some types of cancer. Although prune research for specific human health ben-efits has not been extensive, this fruit's nutritional composition, polyphe-nol content, and popularity as a consumer favorite indicate that research will continue.

Get Dried Plums into Your Diet!

Prunes make a delicious, nutrient- and carbohydrate-enriched snack. Having only a light glycemic effect, they are good sources of calories to sustain energy. The prune is emphasized rather than the fresh plum because it offers easier portability and freedom from having to deal with the juiciness typical of fresh plums. Try a few prunes for snacks or as a side dish at lunch to incorporate this delicious superfruit into your diet. Just four dried plums are one serving.

DRIED PLUM SUPERFRUIT SCORE
Superfruit Score: 12/25
Rank Among 20 Superfruits: 20th
Nutrient Content: 3/5
Phytochemical Content: 3/5
Medical Research Activity: 2/5
Position in Research Pyramid: 1/5
Popularity: 3/5

Superfruits for Life!

Dazzling, wasn't it? From nearly every corner of the world—five continents, four major geographic regions, and at least eight primary countries—common and exotic superfruits are increasingly available in grocery stores near you.

And what is their special interest as *super* fruits? A combination of exceptional nutrient value, phytochemical complexity, and research promise for health benefits from your diet. Think of them as nature's convenient high-nutrient packages that happen to be delicious, inexpensive, portable, and under study by scientists looking for the next breakthroughs in promoting health through whole foods.

If you were to sort through all other fruits known, you'd come upon none with a combination of factors making it as *super* as those of nature's top twenty superfruits!

What we need to cover next is how to shop for them and make these wonderful whole foods regular parts of your diet.

III

Superfruits in Action

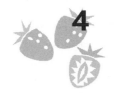

4

Superfruits in Your Shopping Cart

N OW THAT YOU KNOW about the top twenty superfruits and their exceptional nutrient and phytochemical qualities, I'll show you how to shop for them by the Color Code.

I encourage buying fresh fruits, but I'll also explain what product formats are best to look for when buying packaged superfruits. Two tips to always remember are to read the Nutrition Facts panel on packaged goods—it shows you the percentages of daily value (DV) as a nutritional guide—and to scan the list of ingredients that appear in order of how much each was included to manufacture the product. If you have Nutrition Facts, ingredients list, the Color Code, and superfruit signatures in mind every time you shop or have a snack, refreshment, or meal, you'll be well on your way to getting the most nutrition from the foods you eat, creating healthful dietary habits for yourself and your family. That is the key to supercharging your health!

Superfruits and the Color Code

When shopping for superfruits, it's important to think about color, since colors of fruits, as we know, are influenced by specific phytochemical characteristics. Superfruits can be simply cataloged by four color groups as a visual guide for shopping: (1) orange-yellow, (2) red-tan, (3) blue-purple-black, and (4) green. For each shopping trip, meal, or snack, it's easy to use a superfruit Color Code as a way to assure you're getting the most benefits that nature has to share.

Let's think about how the Color Code works. The sections that follow present some easy shopping checklists to help you pick superfruits by their color groups.

Orange-Yellow Superfruits

- ▶ Mango
- ▶ Fig (some varieties)
- ▶ Orange (and other orange-yellow citrus)
- ▶ Goji (wolfberry)
- ▶ Gold kiwifruit
- ▶ Papaya
- ▶ Seaberry

The orange-yellow group is special in that it contains all of the superfruit signatures—prebiotic fiber, vitamin C, provitamin A carotenoids, and polyphenols. Experiment with these fruits to come up with a few you especially like, and then make them routine additions to your diet. Remember that the orange-yellow group is the most powerful for containing all superfruit signatures.

When you see orange and yellow fruits, think "carotenoids" and what they provide as two health values: (1) provitamin A compounds such as beta-carotene, and (2) presumed antioxidant functions of the carotenoid group. Even in green plant foods such as green mango, green guava, kiwifruit, spinach, and broccoli, or red ones like goji and sour cherry, carotenoid content from orange-yellow pigments can be high and yet be concealed by the predominant pigment, green chlorophyll or red anthocyanins.

Great-tasting carotenoid-rich superfruits include mango (orange-yellow-green) varieties in fresh, dried, or 100 percent juice form; any member of the orange family (fresh or as 100 percent juice); papaya (fresh, dried, or 100 percent juice); orange-yellow guava (fresh or 100 percent juice); kiwifruit (fresh, especially the new delicious gold variety); and goji (dried or 100 percent juice).

Red-Tan Superfruits

- Mango
- Fig
- Strawberry
- Goji (wolfberry)
- Red grape
- Cranberry

- Cherry
- Red raspberry
- Red guava
- Pomegranate
- Date

Among these red-tan superfruits, mango (certain cultivars), red guava, and goji contain *both* orange-yellow carotenoids and red anthocyanins. These three superfruits are also hard-to-beat sources of vitamin C and fiber, so they effectively supply the four superfruit signatures.

Blue-Purple-Black Superfruits

- Blueberry
- Blackberry
- Blackcurrant

- Açaí
- Black fig (dried mission variety)
- Dried plum (prune)

Blue-purple-black superfruits are notable for having high contents of three of the primary superfruit signatures: vitamin C, prebiotic fiber, and polyphenols, each fruit having dark blue-purple pigmentation.

The fruits from this list that provide the best sources of vitamin C are blueberries, blackberries, and black figs. Remember that darker fruits usually signify denser nutrient and phytochemical content!

Among my favorite superfruits are blueberries, and I'm especially partial to the size, flavor, and color-richness of wild ("low-bush") blueberries. These pea-size treasures are not always stocked in grocery stores (they are more common in Canada because of the increasing availability of the wild species as frozen produce). Throughout the United States and in British Columbia, cultivation of large highbush blueberries has provided a popular marble-size berry that is firm and juicy, with a richly azure blue skin and blue-green pulp—best experienced in the peak ripening season of July–August. About thirty to fifty fresh blueberries make a succulent low-calorie superfruit snack just by themselves.

Green Superfruits

► Mango (certain cultivars)
► Kiwifruit
► Green guava

Green superfruits get their pigment from likely the most abundant phytochemical—chlorophyll, which may provide benefit by an inhibitory effect on fungi and other environmental toxins. Chlorophyll is also associated with summer green leaves and high-nutrient leafy vegetables such as spinach, romaine, and kale. Green superfruits such as green mango, kiwifruit, and guava are also top sources of vitamin C and prebiotic fiber. Keep in mind that the green pigment in these fruits is predominant and therefore may disguise other pigments present, even red polyphenols or orange-yellow carotenoids.

Think About Superfruit Signatures When Shopping

Given the complex nutrient and phytochemical content of superfruits, it may be too simplistic to say that one or a select few qualities—such as color—stand out as a distinguishing characteristic. Nevertheless, I do think fruit colors are a useful shopping strategy, because colors advertise a superfruit's signatures. Let's look more closely at superfruit signatures to determine which superfruits specifically contain the densest amounts, distinguishing them from the rest.

Of course, all superfruits contain many other nutrients and a complexity of phytochemicals that are comprehensive for overall nutritional value.

Vitamin C

It's a rule of thumb, not an exact science, that bright fruit colors express high vitamin C content. Remember that vitamin C is the fruit's universal antioxidant. Did you know that the density of vitamin C and minerals in a fruit increases as the fruit ripens? During harvest, many fruit growers know that picking fruits at the right time can preserve high levels of vitamin C; you can see this practice reflected by the fresh, bright colors in the grocery store produce section!

As an example, the gold kiwifruit probably represents the best combination of high vitamin C with other superfruit signatures. Give this fascinating, taste-tingling treat a try! You can easily achieve your full daily value of vitamin C by having two to three servings of orange-yellow superfruits. Also, the color red in superfruits almost always means high quantities of polyphenols and vitamin C. Strawberries, red raspberries, cranberries, red guavas, cherries, and goji berries are notable for excellent vitamin C content. The juices from some of these fruits also count for vitamin C content, but the amounts will be lower due to mechanical processing and pasteurization, so be sure to check the Nutrition Facts panel to verify that the product is an excellent source—that is, offering more than 20 percent daily value.

SUPERFRUITS HIGHEST IN VITAMIN C

1. Seaberry
2. Red guava
3. Kiwifruit
4. Blackcurrant
5. Goji (wolfberry)
6. Red raspberry

Prebiotic Fiber

Prebiotic fiber in fruits is most easily associated with pulp—the fleshy, juicy part of a fruit—as opposed to its edible skin or seed coats which provide "insoluble" fiber. Prebiotic fiber provides diversified health benefits supporting advantageous intestinal bacteria and immune functions, all of which help deter both the onset of colon cancer and high blood cholesterol levels.

SUPERFRUITS HIGHEST IN PREBIOTIC FIBER

1. Fig
2. Mango
3. Red raspberry
4. Dried plum (prune)
5. Red guava
6. Goji (wolfberry)

Carotenoids

The phytochemical carotenoids, as previously discussed, are found in orange-yellow superfruits. It's handy to think of carotenoids as indicators of two health values—provitamin A compounds and potential antioxidants.

SUPERFRUITS HIGHEST IN CAROTENOIDS

1. Seaberry
2. Mango
3. Papaya
4. Goji (wolfberry)
5. Gold kiwifruit
6. Orange

Polyphenols

When you see mouthwatering red, blue, purple, or black fruits, you can be sure there are polyphenols present. The highest-density polyphenols are most likely from anthocyanin pigments embedded in the skins or rinds of fruits, but polyphenols also include members of the general flavonoid group such as quercetin, catechin, gallic acid, and ellagic acid, which have been linked to a variety of possible health benefits, among them being lowered risk of cancer.

You probably know of this class of phytochemicals already, as polyphenols are the main reasons the superfruit industry started. For years, it was assumed that polyphenols are dietary antioxidants, but this role is now doubted by scientists. Instead, a new theory is that polyphenols have other important functions in promoting health, such as fine-tuning of enzymes, genes, receptors, and proteins, some of which may be the "on-off" switches for diseases—especially chronic inflammation thought to be common as an onset mediator of numerous diseases.

SUPERFRUITS HIGHEST IN POLYPHENOLS

1. Cranberry
2. Blueberry
3. Blackberry
4. Blackcurrant
5. Red raspberry
6. Red grape

Superfruit Formats and Retail Brands

Although eating the fresh fruit is the preferred way to consume your superfruits, there will be times when the convenience of retail packaged products holds sway. You may get meaningful clues about the Color Code with certain packaged superfruit products, but most often you will have to read the ingredients list and Nutrition Facts panel. You can promptly spot three of the superfruit signatures among the Nutrition Facts: vitamin A (from provitamin A carotenoids), vitamin C, and dietary fiber, which all should be in excess of 10 percent daily value (the "good" content level; above 20 percent DV is "excellent"). Let's discover how to navigate through the blizzard of superfruit products in retail or Internet channels.

Superfruits in Smoothies

Bottled smoothies present a custom-made format for manufacturers to combine superfruits with nutrient fortification. The creamy, heavy texture of a smoothie often lends itself to reestablishing the dietary fiber content of a product. Although you will be greeted by a wide variety of products in this category, the global firm Nestlé, two major American brands—Bolthouse Farms and Odwalla, and Arthur's Fresh Company, in Canada, provide examples among their numerous products that preserve the most nutrients from the fresh fruit. Here's a rundown:

► **Bolthouse Farms Berry Boost** (bolthouse.com)—contains blueberries, boysenberries (related to raspberries and blackberries), red raspberries, blackberries, and strawberries; fortified with vitamin C and dietary fiber

► **Bolthouse Farms C Goodness**—contains mango and acerola (a tree fruit that is one of the emerging superfruits and is a natural highly enriched source of vitamin C); fortified with the antioxidant A-C-E vitamins

► **Bolthouse Farms Blue Goodness**—contains blueberries, blackberries, and elderberries (see Appendix C); fortified with vitamins C and K and dietary fiber

- **Odwalla Blueberry B** (odwalla.com)—contains orange juice, blueberry puree, mango puree, banana puree, and Concord grape juice; fortified with vitamin C and seven B vitamins
- **Odwalla C Monster**—contains orange juice, peach puree, apple juice, guava puree, pineapple juice, acerola juice, and raspberry puree; fortified with ten times the daily value for vitamin C (from the acerola) and vitamin K
- **Arthur's Fresh Company POMtastic** (arthursjuice.com)—contains pomegranate juice, apple juice, banana puree, and blackcurrant puree; fortified with dietary fiber, vitamins C, D, and E, five B vitamins, and three dietary minerals
- **Nestlé Boost** (nestle-nutrition.com)—superfruit *flavored* products (strawberry, raspberry) sold as a nutritional energy drink fortified with an impressive array of added nutrients

Superfruits as 100 Percent Pure Juices

Superfruit juices that contain 100 percent pure juices have nutrient value, but generally, these juices don't live up to the overall nutritional value of the whole, fresh fruit. Among makers of numerous 100 percent juice products, major brands such as Tropicana and Minute Maid are usually the easiest ones to find:

- **Tropicana** (tropicana.com)—makes fifteen varieties of 100 percent juices from oranges and other citrus and superfruits, some blended and fortified with vitamin C, calcium, omega fats, or extra pulp (fiber)
- **Minute Maid** (minutemaid.com)—has several 100 percent juice products and a group of drinks called "enhanced" juices, which contain added vitamins and other essential nutrients; Enhanced Pomegranate Blueberry Flavored 100% Juice contains apple, grape, pomegranate, blueberry, and raspberry juices and is fortified with an algae oil for omega fats, vitamins C, E, and B_{12}, and soy lecithin

Superfruits in Yogurts

One of the choice formats for providing fruits and extra nutrients is yogurt, either as a creamy, stirred skim or soy milk eaten with a spoon or as one of the increasingly popular drinkable yogurts, which are loved especially by kids.

In both instances, the product is usually cooled throughout storage, an important parameter that allows cultures of "good" bacteria to be added. This is the best format for getting your *probiotic* food value from fruit products (*probiotic* means that it contains added healthful bacteria to complement the billions already existing in your intestinal system). Two major manufacturers offer products worth sampling:

▶ **Stony Field FarmWild Berry Smoothie** (stonyfield.com)—a yogurt containing juices from blueberries and beets (for extra anthocyanins) plus five B vitamins and other essential nutrients
▶ **Silk Soymilk** products (silksoymilk.com)—include blueberry, raspberry, cherry, and strawberry juice/puree in nutrient-fortified soy milk yogurt with six active cultures

Superfruits in Granola Bars

This popular and versatile product format containing superfruits has considerable diversity among manufacturers. Two major producers are Odwalla (again) and Nature's Path, the latter an organic-only manufacturer whose products may be more expensive:

▶ **Odwalla Berries GoMega Bar**—contains a blend of purees from figs, dates, and berries, plus flaxseeds, soy meal, and sunflower oil
▶ **Nature's Path PomegranCherry Optimum Energy Bar** (natures path.com/products/bars)—among many grain and seed ingredients, contains date puree, pomegranate juice concentrate, raisins, dried cherries, freeze-dried raspberry pieces, red beet juice concentrate (for extra anthocyanins), and vitamin E; it is rich in dietary fiber and essential minerals

Superfruits in Breakfast Cereals

There's wisdom in fortifying breakfast cereals: many consumers pay more attention to this first meal of the day than others, and many also use cereals for snacks. Aware of these habits, manufacturers have recently begun to really stack simple cereals with extra nutrients. This is a positive trend also accounting for the growing use of freeze-dried berries and other fruit pieces in cereals. Here are two examples:

▶ **Kellogg's Special K Blueberry Cereal** (specialk.com/#/products)— provides whole grains with dried blueberry pieces and puree in a cereal fortified with excellent percentages of daily values for dietary fiber, vitamins A, C, and D, six B vitamins, and four essential minerals; other superfruits featured are strawberry, raisin, cranberry, and elderberry in cereals or nutrition bars

▶ **General Mills Berry Burst, Triple Berry Cheerios** (generalmills .com)—takes advantage of the FDA-recognized health benefit regarding the ability of whole-oat products to provide a cholesterol-lowering effect from prebiotic fiber; this simple cereal favored by generations of kids continues to deliver on many nutrients— excellent levels of vitamins A, C, and D, six B vitamins, and several essential minerals in the familiar O's, combined with dried strawberries, red raspberries, and blueberries

Superfruits in Packaged Products

For some consumers, fruits packaged in cans or plastic bowls are a convenient option. Two companies with familiar products that have been popular over decades are Del Monte and Dole. Both have jumped into the superfruits arena with new promotional campaigns:

▶ **Del Monte** (delmonte.com)—offers the traditional fruit cocktail now in a "Carb-Clever" product that uses Splenda as a zero-calorie sweetener and contains a high level of vitamin C; in 2008, Del Monte launched a "Try Superfruits" campaign featuring packaged products trademarked Superfruit snacks, which include mango, orange, blackberry, pomegranate, and açaí (trysuperfruit.com)

▶ **Dole** (dolesuperfoods.com)—has assembled a group of "Superfood" products containing many superfruits linked to potential health benefits for individual organs or systems, including heart, eyes, brain, antioxidants, skin, joints, bones, immune system, and prostate gland

---

MOST EXOTIC SUPERFRUITS

In recognition that the superfruit category is still becoming known among the public, I want to give you a handful of five fruits to try that may be relatively unfamiliar and yet provide loads of taste, convenience of format, and a combination of superfruit signature qualities for nutrients and phytochemicals:

1. Mango—fresh, frozen, or as a juice; among the wide variety available as fresh produce, my favorites are the gold, kidney-shaped Alphonso and Ataulfo
2. Gold kiwifruit—fresh
3. Red guava—fresh; the "strawberry" guava probably sports the widest-appealing taste, fragrance, and color among the many varieties
4. Figs—fresh or dried; explore for your favorite (dried black mission figs are a real eating pleasure and contain good levels of polyphenols; dried gold Turkish figs are also a nutrient-rich treat). Dried figs have better portability and are a pleasant chewing experience likely having the most appeal across age groups.
5. Dates—pitted-dried; explore for your favorite (Deglet Noor is an inexpensive, low-sugar cultivar that is appealing to eat and high in nutritional value)

Less Common Superfruits: Goji (Wolfberry), Seaberry, and Açaí

From the list of nature's top twenty superfruits, goji, seaberry, and açaí are three that are exotic and perhaps the most difficult to obtain in whole-fruit form. However, other product formats are becoming increasingly popular.

Goji (Wolfberry). Goji berries are commercially grown in China and may be sold regionally there as fresh, but they are not exported fresh. You can get them as dried berries—having a consistency like that of dry raisins—from specialty fruit shops in Chinatowns of the United States, Canada, and Europe, or through websites. The nutrient analyses of dried goji berries show an exceptionally rich and diverse content, so give them a try for a no-hassle, nourishing snack!

In the following list is information about different formats for goji products. In addition to the dried berry, you may wish to try juice concentrate, powder preparations, or confectionery products, which will have lower nutritional value. Here are a few online stores:

▶ **Rich Nature Nutraceutical Labs** (richnature.com/onlinestore)— organic- and kosher-certified (implying the farm and processing facilities have been inspected to assure no use of pesticides and high standards for authenticity and quality of the fruit) juice concentrate, plain dried organic- and kosher-certified berries, chocolate- or yogurt-covered dried organic- and kosher-certified berries, seed oil soap
▶ **St. Francis Herb Farm** (stfrancisherbfarm.com)—dried berries, 100 percent juice
▶ **Navitas Naturals** (navitasnaturals.com)—dried organic- and kosher-certified berries, pulp powder
▶ **Absolutefruitz** (absolutefruitz.com)—juices including goji, pomegranate, blueberry, mulberry, and tropical fruits; Absolute Red organic juice/puree, seed oil dispenser, and organic-certified dried berries (absolute-red.com)

Seaberry (Sea buckthorn). Intrepid consumers may come across fresh or frozen berries from artisan outlets in southern Canada, but otherwise this superfruit is not grown on a commercial scale in North America and is not widely imported, so it is rare in American stores. Seaberry products are popular in a variety of fresh, dried, beverage, and kitchen products in northern Europe, Russia, India, and Southeast Asia.

Because of the high content of omega fats in both the pulp and seeds, seaberries have become a popular botanical cosmetic resource for skin creams, shampoos, soap, lip balm, and spa oils. Some people prefer taking oil capsules for the possible benefit of omega fatty acids from seaberry pulp or seeds. You can also put your taste buds to the test for the unusual tart flavor of seaberry by trying juice or powder products. Here are some selected purveyors:

- **Rich Nature Nutraceutical Labs** (richnature.com/onlinestore)—juice powder, pulp oil dispenser, seed oil capsules
- **Seabuckthorn International** (seabuckthorn.com)—cleansing bars, shampoo and conditioner, fruit extract, pulp and seed oil capsules and dispensers, skin cream, lip balm and gloss, tea
- **Sibu** (sibu.com)—juice blend, tea, seed and pulp oil capsules, soap, skin cream, equine products
- **Christine Berger GmbH and Sandokan** (sandokan.de)—some fifty edible offerings, including multiple juice, candy, jam, liquor, wine, salad dressing, and nutrition bar products

Açaí. Commercial development of açaí berries is still evolving. Because special handling requirements and other factors prevent the fruit's exportation as fresh or frozen whole berries, açaí is likely to be seen only as a juice, puree, pulp powder, or pulp oil on global markets in the foreseeable future. Açaí has become popular for its coloring and flavoring properties and exotic origin from the Amazon. The pulp powder is best for smoothie product applications containing the natural high nutrient profile, but juices, with lower nutritional value often blended with other fruits, are already popular. Here are some shopping possibilities:

- **Sambazon** (sambazon.com)—bottled organic smoothies, organic juices, organic powder packs, sorbets, capsules
- **Arthur's Fresh Company** (arthursjuice.com)—Açaí Plus contains purees of açaí berries, blackberries, blueberries, and boysenberries, apple and pear juices, and banana puree; fortified with dietary fiber, antioxidant A-C-E vitamins, and nine other essential nutrients
- **Navitas Naturals** (navitasnaturals.com)—organic and kosher certified pulp powder
- **Universal Taste** (universaltaste.com)—organic sorbets, frozen pulp, freeze-dried pulp
- **Bolthouse Farms** (bomdia.com)—Bomdia, a delicious sweetened juice

▶ **Superfruit Oils** (superfruitoils.com)—pure pulp oil for food, cosmetic, and capsule applications

Best Frozen Superfruits

▶ Blueberry
▶ Red grape
▶ Kiwifruit

▶ Cherry
▶ Cranberry
▶ Mango

As a convenience, many manufacturers and distributors are packaging superfruits as frozen whole fruit or cut pieces. Analyses of nutritional contents show that frozen fruits preserve nutrients closely to those of fresh or dried fruits, so this is an acceptable format that may be more suitable to some people, especially those with limited access to fresh markets or out-of-season produce.

Best-Bang-for-Your-Buck Superfruits

The entries in the following list present my top ten suggestions for obtaining the best ratio of nutrient value to cost. All are best as fresh whole fruits except fig, blackcurrant, and plum (prune), which are more commonly available and versatile in dried form:

1. Navel orange
2. Date
3. Dried fig
4. Red grape
5. Mango

6. Dried plum (prune)
7. Dried blackcurrant
8. Strawberry
9. Cherry
10. Kiwifruit

Think of these superfruits as the ones from which you could get the most nutritional benefit if budget were an issue. Remember that whole fresh oranges contain all four superfruit signatures in high concentration, in addition to being refreshing to eat and inexpensive, so make an effort to eat one a day. Save the peel for a variety of other nutrient, flavoring, and fragrance uses. Dates are a nutrient-dense, high-calorie food, probably the least expensive fruit per unit of weight on this list. Dried figs, red grapes (and raisins), dried plums, dried blackcurrants, strawberries, cherries, and kiwifruit are wonderful-tasting, highly nutritious fruits, diverse in portability and uses, and relatively inexpensive compared with other, nonnutritious snack products. And finally, the mango—the top-ranked superfruit—can be eaten fresh as it is (often very juicy!) or as dried slices (versatile, portable, and tasty!). It would be a meal with great taste and nutrient impact just by itself.

Additional Tips

Adopting superfruits for your diet is a *dedication to your health*—it should be a daily reminder to abstain from unhealthful fast foods and other overprocessed carbohydrates, high-fat dairy products, and high-sugar beverages. To get the most out of nature's top twenty superfruits, you should aim to have *at least three different colors* of superfruits in your basket when grocery shopping. Ask your produce section grocer what he or she recommends that day.

Remember to choose the most brightly colored fruits and make a stop at the store's bulk section to stock up on dried fruits, whole grains, nuts, and seeds. Buying in bulk almost always is cheaper. You will notice that the produce and bulk bin sections of the grocery store are usually near the front of the store, making it even easier to start and end your shopping trip with the superfruits you need.

Finally, always scan the Nutrition Facts panel on product labels of any packaged goods you consider buying. Note the *absence* of nutrients and the high caloric contents of many packaged foods or beverages. When you compare those items with what you can put into your body using fresh, dried, or frozen superfruits, you will convince yourself that you can easily supply nutrient density with fabulous-tasting *whole-food* superfruits. By achieving this stage, you put yourself on a path to healthier living and lifelong wellness. Superfruits are a vehicle carrying you to better health, so get on board!

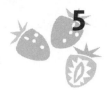

Superfruits in Your Daily Diet

B ECAUSE OF THE NUTRIENT richness of superfruits, using them regularly will help create a daily diet that is economical as well as easier
and more enjoyable as you grow familiar with the variety of choices for
nutrient profile, flavor, and color. Just three servings per day can bolster
overall health! I limit the lists for each superfruit group in this chapter to
just a few having the best combination of nutrient content, taste, simplicity, and affordability, but you should try different superfruit choices to
develop your own favorites. I'll also show you how to include superfruits
in a healthy meal plan: the Mediterranean diet.

Superfruits with Breakfast

Your goal should be to involve whole fruits in your meals from the beginning of each day. Whole-grain bread or cereal with pieces of superfruits
would be ideal. Simply heat up a bowl of oatmeal, add some low-calorie
yogurt fortified with vitamin D and omega fats, toss in a few pieces of
your favorite superfruit, and enjoy. Now you're ready to tackle the morning. Refer to Chapter 6 for breakfast recipes and smoothie recipes, which
are *super* ways to launch yourself into the day.

Try these in oatmeal, with yogurt, or by themselves:

- ► Fresh or frozen berries of any kind
- ► Date slices
- ► Dried goji berries (wolfberries), cranberries, raisins,
  or blackcurrants
- ► Pieces of dried figs

Oatmeal is the easiest food preparation for getting the "fiber effect": eating fiber-rich foods containing beta-glucan polysaccharides (the prebiotic fiber of whole grains credited by the FDA with lowering the risk of some cancers and cardiovascular diseases), as oatmeal does, can reduce your blood cholesterol count within a few weeks of daily use—a benefit claim approved by the FDA. Mixing oatmeal with superfruits, yogurt, and seeds or nuts is a simple way to start your mornings with a nutrient and phytochemical burst consisting of fiber, protein, omega fats, provitamin A carotenoids, polyphenols, and multiple micronutrients.

Best Superfruits for Jams, Preserves, or Marmalades

▶ Wild blueberry
▶ Blackberry
▶ Orange and other citrus
▶ Seaberry
▶ Blackcurrant

Jams, preserves, and marmalades can be spread on whole-grain bread, added to oatmeal, or used as dessert toppings. I put thin slices of orange and lemon peel in my blueberry jam for extra flavor and nutrient value! Orange-grapefruit-lemon-lime marmalades can be fortified with extra pieces from your stored peels.

Seaberry jams with marzipan, berry pieces, pineapple, and orange peel are popular in Europe. Jams, jellies, and salad dressings offer familiar formats for getting to know the nutrient-dense but tart-tasting seaberry. Blackcurrant jam, for its part, contributes that unique mild bitterness resulting from its intense vitamin C and polyphenol contents—a reminder about the superfruit signatures inside.

Superfruits with Lunch and Dinner

The way to optimize these nutrient-rich sources in your daily meals is to make them an *essential* part of *every* meal and snack. You don't need all twenty superfruits in your kitchen, but only a few of your favorites daily—to keep variety of interest—and then only a serving of each for main courses, desserts, and snacks. To get your five to ten total daily servings of colorful fruits and vegetables, this is easy, isn't it?

There are several ways to pair superfruits with lunch and dinner. Why not try including some in a whole-grain bread wrap with fresh vegetables? You can also sauté fish or meats and use superfruits as a topping or side dish. Some combination of superfruits giving two to three servings would be an asset to any meal. And remember the general rule that a superfruit serving is an amount that would fit in the palm of your hand.

Side Dishes

- ► Sliced gold or green kiwifruit
- ► Fresh or dried mango chunks
- ► Large cultivated blueberries
- ► Pitted fresh sweet cherries
- ► Fresh blackberries

By serving the superfruit as a side dish, you can also eliminate dessert, saving that tempting calorie count. The superfruit choices will vary according to taste and appearance preferences, but wouldn't two or three of the five listed here be inviting enough to include beside your typical plate of food?

Sauces with Fish or Meats

- ► Cranberry
- ► Seaberry
- ► Blackcurrant
- ► Mango
- ► Orange

Integrate berry sauces in your main meals regularly, rather than enjoying them just twice a year between Thanksgiving and New Year's Eve. Each of these superfruits provides a color-rich, tangy sauce complement for practically any hot dish, meat, or dessert. Scan the recipes in Chapter 6 for ideas on making superfruit compotes and sauces.

Fresh Vegetable Salads

- ► Blueberries
- ► Red raspberries
- ► Mandarin or navel orange slices with pith and peel slices

- ▶ Goji berries (wolfberries)
- ▶ Sliced Medjool dates (*Medjool* means "unknown" cultivar; these have a higher moisture content and more sugar than Deglet Noor)

Pieces of colorful crisp or chewy fruit among your favorite vegetable greens add nutrition, taste, and visual interest for livelier, high-nutrient salads. For tossed salads, I look for differences in taste, color, and juice content to play against the more bland lettuce or spinach greens, beans, red cabbage, and tomatoes. These standard ingredients are nutritious plant foods in themselves, but I often feel such a salad needs more color and nutrient content, which you can get from superfruits.

How about adding roasted unsalted pumpkin or sunflower seeds, walnuts, and a few superfruit pieces to your salad? Blueberries and red raspberries speak for themselves; with their pleasing colors, juice, and one-of-a-kind tastes, you can hardly wait to get the refreshing nuggets on your fork.

You can also use luscious, bite-size mandarins for color and sweetness, or cut up a navel orange, keeping as much fiber-rich pith and limonene-loaded peel as you like. I use mandarins often and add a few squirts of orange, lemon, or lime juice to shower the whole salad! Don't forget the date: salads are light eating, of course, but you can fortify yours even more with nutrient, taste, and calorie value by tossing in slices of this mellow-tasting, sweet, chewy superfruit!

Superfruits on the Fly! Super Snacks

In the typical Western diet, snacking is one of the main culprits in the "crime" of consuming calories empty of nutrients. Doughnuts, chips, cookies, fat-filled muffins, bleached or sugared bagels, and sweetened rolls are all calorie-laden, overprocessed fillers devoid of nutrients. Let's change to healthier habits: I recommend turning to three of your favorite superfruits, either fresh or dried, whenever you crave a snack.

The dried superfruits highlighted in this section are best for on-the-go snacks and are readily found in bulk bins. They are inexpensive, simple solutions for getting a combination of high nutrient value; low glycemic load; a pleasant, natural, sweet taste; and enjoyable chewing. Mixing a few together in two handfuls is really all you need for a mid-morning or afternoon energy boost. That's right: two handfuls of dried superfruits will give you two servings toward your daily fruit intake!

Best Superfruits for *Dried* Eating

- Dates
- Figs
- Red grapes (as raisins)

- Goji berries (wolfberries)
- Cranberries
- Blackcurrants

The convenience factor of dried superfruit finger foods makes this category of nutrient-rich fruits all the more convincing for anyone's diet. I want to promote the simplicity factor for helping readers of this book appreciate how easy it is to follow wise dietary plans using inexpensive superfruits—and these six fruits meet that requirement!

As relatively large dried fruits, whole dates and figs can be tapped for any occasion. Keeping dates or figs nearby (in a ziplock bag for freshness and to prevent stickiness) makes it a snap to get your superfruit servings each day—whether around the home for a snack or on the go.

With raisins as your point of reference, you may find dried goji berries, cranberries, or blackcurrants tasty and trouble-free side dishes or snacks. Mixing these four together with a few walnuts, almonds, and unsalted roasted pumpkin seeds produces a flavorful, multicolored, nutrient-dense medley! Remember that dried fruits are also an inspired way to incorporate superfruits for lunch or dinner—just sprinkle a handful on your plate with any main dish!

High-Energy Granola or Trail Mixes

- Dates
- Dried figs
- Dried goji berries (wolfberries)

- Dried plums (prunes)
- Dried blackcurrants

Some granolas and trail mixes have a loose composition of whole-grain flakes (usually oats), seeds, nuts, and dried fruit. For these, dates, dried figs, goji berries, and/or dried blackcurrants are just the thing to add either individually or together. Other cereal mixes can be made with a half tablespoon of molasses, honey, or berry syrup to stick everything together in a bar or cake. Dates, dried figs, and prunes cut into nibble-size chunks—typically sticky themselves—lend themselves well to making the granola ingredients stick together for portability, desirable nutrient density, and satisfying taste.

Mixed-Fruit Salads

▶ Fresh red raspberries or blackberries
▶ Mango chunks
▶ Mandarin or navel oranges (sectioned, sliced with pith and peel); blood oranges
▶ Fresh red or black grapes (with seeds for extra crunch appeal and nutrient content)
▶ Papaya chunks

I relish red raspberries and blackberries; they are high on the list because their delicate texture, beautiful color, exceptional prebiotic fiber content, and slight sourness can really set a fruit salad apart with distinct freshness. Some people may be dissuaded by the crunch of seeds from these two *Rubus* berries, but the seeds impart a little tartness and are loaded with micronutrients, so you know you're getting extra nutrition from them.

Among the important new nutrients discussed in Part I is a group of cholesterol-lowering phytosterols, which are concentrated most in seeds. The seeds of black grapes and dried or fresh figs are two excellent examples.

Mango and fresh or dried papaya chunks add tropical flavor and color to a fruit salad, and either can star as the main fruit of a mixed salad. You need only a few bite-size chunks of either fruit to get a lip-smacking dose of nutrients. For extra fiber intake, leave the mango's skin on the sections you cut; it's usually thin, chewy, and mostly tasteless, making it an easy solution for getting more fiber and pigments.

For mixed-fruit salads, try mandarins—those smaller, sweeter oranges that make neatly sized segments for the spoon or fork. As horticulture adds new cultivars for consumers to try, look for oranges with deeper colors of red or even purple, usually called "blood" oranges or cara cara. These varieties have even higher carotenoid (provitamin A and/or lycopene) and anthocyanin contents, giving them richer pigmentation and thereby adding superfruit signatures we want. The red-pulp oranges have a mellow flavor, almost like mango or papaya.

Salsas

- Mangoes
- Oranges
- Dates
- Cranberries
- Blueberries

Why not nutritious fruits in salsa? Small amounts of dried, fresh, or pureed superfruits in your favorite spicy salsa contribute extra nutrients, texture, color, and interest. For purees, just toss a few pieces into your blender, and pulse for a few seconds to get the texture you prefer. Try the superfruits listed here to give extra fun to dipping with whole-grain chips or breads.

Superfruits with Desserts

- Dates
- Dried figs
- Dried plums (prunes)
- Oranges
- Red grape raisins
- Dried goji berries

A time will come when you have that yearning for something sweet. What do you reach for: a candy bar, or a nutrient-rich fruit with satisfying sugar content? I hope this book encourages you to satisfy your sweet cravings with great-tasting superfruits! Dates, dried figs, dried plums, oranges, raisins, or goji berries are all you need for a sweet-tooth treat. A bowl containing two each of dates, figs, and prunes plus a medium-size navel orange cut into eight segments and a handful of raisins—and maybe another handful of sunflower seeds—would take care of that yearning in no time.

Other possibilities are dried mango slices, fresh strawberries, red grapes, whole kiwifruit, blueberries, fresh or dried sweet cherries, dried blackcurrants, and a fresh, crisp Red Delicious apple or a pear. For a wholesome dip, use triple-fruit marmalade with extra rind; whole-fruit blueberry, blackcurrant, or strawberry jam.

If you are able to buy dried goji berries (wolfberries) at a good price, include them—there's something about goji that is mysteriously filling (likely related to its high prebiotic fiber content from the goji's dense content of polysaccharides). Just seventy dried berries or twenty grams (about 0.4 ounce)—a generous one-serving handful—takes care of my yearnings for sweets, and, all the while, I know I am getting high nutrient impact from such a simple snack.

Chocolate Fondues and Chocolate-Covered Superfruits

▶ Large cultivated blueberries ▶ Dried figs

▶ Deglet Noor dates ▶ Strawberries

▶ Sweet pitted cherries ▶ Dried plums (prunes)

There is an undeniable pleasure to be enjoyed from warmed chocolate combined with fresh fruit. The six fruits listed are irresistible targets for impaling on a long fondue fork and dipping into melted chocolate.

There is growing acceptance among nutrition experts that occasionally eating dark chocolate containing a high percentage of cocoa provides polyunsaturated fats and flavonoids that may benefit cognitive abilities during aging, as well as anti-inflammatory and anticlotting effects, among other potential health benefits still being analyzed in research. So, the combination of superfruits and chocolate may be both healthy and delicious! Eat chocolate treats in moderate amounts so you can have fun without guilt!

Super Health: Superfruits and the Mediterranean Diet

You may be asking yourself, "Where do whole superfruits fit in a healthy dietary plan such as the Mediterranean diet?" Many of nature's top twenty superfruits are in fact native to the Mediterranean region—and are commonly available, making them typical additions for meals and snacks throughout the day. These Mediterranean fruits are fresh and dried figs, oranges, strawberries, red grapes, bilberries (European "blueberries"), cherries, red raspberries, blackberries, dates, and pomegranates—that's half of the top twenty superfruits!

The Mediterranean diet is not a weight-loss plan or a fad but rather has a substantial scientific basis adopted by numerous public health experts, nutrition strategists, and governments around the world in their efforts to establish healthful eating habits. Where practiced over decades in countries bordering the Mediterranean Sea, the Mediterranean diet has been shown to extend adult life expectancy to the highest in the world and to lower rates of coronary heart disease, certain cancers, and other diet-related chronic diseases. It is part of a lifestyle that includes regular physical activity leading to healthier body weights and lower rates of metabolic syndrome (obesity, diabetes) than elsewhere among developed countries.

The Mediterranean diet is characterized by abundant use of plant foods (fruits, vegetables, whole grain breads, other forms of cereals, beans, nuts, and seeds), fresh fruit as the typical main-meal side dish and daily dessert, olive oil as the principal source of fat on salads and breads, low amounts of dairy products (principally cheese and yogurt), and fish or poultry as meats used in low to moderate frequency. Water is the usual beverage, but also red wine—for which there is ample research indicating cardiovascular health benefits—is consumed in low to moderate amounts, normally with the evening meal.

A Mediterranean Diet Including Superfruits: General Guide

Emphasized throughout this book is a whole-food diet that includes superfruits to simplify and optimize nutrient content in formats enjoyable to eat. An outline of such a Mediterranean-like dietary plan looks like this:

Mediterranean diet food group	Servings
Whole fruits and vegetables	5–7 daily
Superfruits	3–5 daily contributing to the entry above
Whole-grain breads, pasta, cereals	3–5 daily
Legumes (beans)	1–2 daily
Seeds, nuts	1–2 daily
Fish	3–5 per week—salmon, mackerel, sardines
Cooking and salad oils	Daily use of olive, canola, soy, sesame, or sunflower oil
Red wine	1 glass with afternoon or evening meals
Water	Frequently throughout the day (the primary beverage)
Poultry, lean red meats	1–2 per week or none; or substituted with soy products
Eggs, dairy foods	3 per week or none; or substituted with soy products

Benefits of a Mediterranean Diet Including Whole Superfruits

My proposal here is that you adopt the strongest scientific support for a regular diet providing health benefits—the Mediterranean diet—combined with all the advantages of superfruits. Here's how it works:

▶ Provides delicious food choices well supported by current medical and epidemiological (population) research for extending life and reducing disease risk
▶ Emphasizes extraordinary nutrient content and high phytochemical content and is well supported by extensive medical research
▶ Promotes benefits of high-fiber fruits and prebiotic fiber for general digestive health
▶ Conforms to 2008 health advisories and dietary recommendations entitled "Fruits and Veggies—More Matters" by the U.S. government's leading health agencies: Department of Health and Human Services, National Institutes of Health, National Cancer Institute, and Centers for Disease Control and Prevention

- Beyond the sixteen countries of the Mediterranean basin, principles of the Mediterranean diet are adopted as national nutrition policy by the United Nations, World Health Organization, and more than thirty developed countries.

Tips for Including Superfruits in a Mediterranean Diet

Once you understand the food groups of the Mediterranean diet, it's easy to insert superfruits into daily practice. Here are a few ideas:

- Meals are not about calorie quantity, but rather *nutrient quantity and quality*—with lower overall food (and therefore calorie) intake made simple by using whole-food superfruits.
- Of course, you do not need *all* superfruits in your diet every week. From the top twenty, use three every day for a week in snacks or meals each day; then change among your favorites. This plan is intended to be simple, readily achievable, and inexpensive. So, no excuses!
- Eating three or more servings of superfruits every day is all that's needed for baseline nutrient intake. Add to that two servings of differently colored vegetables or other fruits, and you have met your minimal fruit and vegetable intake quota.
- Not counting your protein portion of fish or extra-firm tofu, have at least three different colors of superfruits *and* vegetables or other fruits on *every* meal plate.
- Include at least two superfruits in every garden salad.
- Keep your fresh and dried superfruits visible in your house. Encourage kids to eat from that supply first before considering any other snack.
- Use seeds and nuts liberally with your superfruit servings; these are high-nutrient food sources rich in mono- and polyunsaturated heart-healthy fats, and they go together well with fruit!
- As much as your taste allows, use colorful, rich spices as a sprinkling on sauces or meals prepared in a pot, such as pasta and tomato sauce. Curry powder, turmeric, cumin, and cayenne pepper, for example, not only lend terrific flavors and pleasant colors but also

are rich in polyphenols shown in research to potentially benefit health, often by virtue of the same phytochemicals as are in super-fruits. Believe me, spices go fine with cooked, fresh, or dried super-fruits in those same meals—especially cinnamon on oatmeal with your superfruits.

▶ Use olive or canola oil as a base for every stir-fry or salad dressing, or even as the dressing itself. Canola is less expensive than olive oil and equally balanced in desirable heart-healthy fats. Sprinkle dried superfruits into your stir-fry for extra nutrients, taste, and visual appeal.

▶ When you feel your first sense of fullness at a main meal, stop eating and push the plate away. This way, you limit calorie intake and save room for the superfruit dessert!

▶ Finish every main meal with a whole-superfruit dessert. Include lots of variety throughout the week. Add nuts and seeds for extra nutrients and enjoyment.

Now that we have a framework for using superfruits in the Mediterranean diet, let's move on to the recipes to see the variety of ways to include superfruits regularly in your diet!

Superfruit Recipes

I N THIS FINAL CHAPTER, I will show you how superfruits can be con-venient and inexpensive nutrient sources in your diet. Getting back to those old-fashioned skills of preparing your meals at home—and maybe even some superfruit home-gardening—would help you stretch your food budget and get the most nutritional bang for your buck.

One purpose in choosing this chapter's recipes was to encourage simplicity. I will be giving you ideas for fruit preparations using common procedures and tools—keeping it basic, with minimal fuss. Maybe you will recognize some traditional or even nostalgic dishes that you know and love, with the slight twist of just adding a fruit or two that may be unfamiliar to you. These are healthful, nutrient-packed options that even your kids can love!

Remember that whole foods should be your first choice for meals and snacks, as they represent the best ways available for maximizing nutri-tional health and enhancing disease prevention through what we eat. *Whole-food* fruits, vegetables, grains, nuts, and seeds provide the opti-mal range and density of nutrients that contribute to reducing the risk of cardiovascular disease and several types of cancer. You'll see that my recipes easily combine superfruits into various whole-food meals that can supercharge your health!

In the following sections, you'll find recipes for six preparations:

▶ Smoothies
▶ Breakfast and snacks
▶ Salads

▶ Sauces
▶ Seafood entrees
▶ Desserts

Other than for smoothies, each recipe includes a Superfruit Recipe Snapshot, which gives you information about nutrient and phytochemical content, as well as a superfruit Color Code designation.

For a few recipes, I'll also suggest possible superfruit substitutes—so, take these as hints and be flexible to mix, match, or swap superfruit ingredients that appeal to your own taste!

KITCHEN CONVERSIONS

Nutrition Facts panels on product packages are based on one serving size (which varies according to food) or on 100 grams, which equals 3.5 ounces, or 0.44 U.S. cup.

1 U.S. cup = 8 ounces = 240 milliliters

1 U.S. tablespoon = 0.5 ounce = 15 milliliters

$°C = (°F − 32) × 0.56$

$°F = °C × 1.8 + 32$

Smoothies

Prepared with a conventional blender, my smoothie recipes have several common features:

▶ **Fortified soy milk rather than dairy milk.** I choose fortified soy products because they have higher contents of micronutrients, heart-healthy omega fats, sterols, and a polyphenol class called isoflavones, which also may be beneficial. These features are not present comparatively in dairy milk. Protein and carbohydrate levels are about the same between soy and dairy milks, but adequate content of these macronutrients is supplied by the superfruits you choose. Also, if you are fond of vanilla, as I am, most brands of soy milk include a vanilla-flavored product that goes well with fruits.

▶ **Low-fat or nonfat yogurt.** I also prefer vanilla-flavored yogurt for a neutral taste with a little extra vanilla flavor, which suits most smoothies. You can also use frozen low-fat yogurt in place of ice cream.

▶ **Flaxseeds.** I add whole flaxseeds by the handful to almost every smoothie to get three qualities: extra micronutrients and fiber, a little burst of the nutlike taste of flaxseeds, and a crunchy texture. Experiment—or add your own seed or nut favorite!

▶ **Splenda rather than granulated sugar for sweetening.** Some superfruits have a mild to moderate sourness, especially from their skins, a result of those desirable phytochemicals—polyphenolic acids—that give color to fruits and vegetables and are reputed to be antioxidants. To compensate for that sourness, Splenda provides a *zero-calorie*, high-sweetness impact in a small amount, is quickly soluble, and is barely noticed in a blended smoothie. Present in hundreds of consumer products, Splenda is a safe, effective alternative to sugar.

▶ **Ripe bananas and pineapple juice.** Though these two fruits are not mentioned in the industry as superfruits (they should be, in my opinion), bananas and pineapple juice are nevertheless inexpensive and agreeable companions for almost every smoothie. If you like their taste, use them often for the bonus of natural sweetness, extra nutrients, and versatility in recipes. If you use pineapple juice in your smoothie recipe, you probably won't need any other sweetener.

▶ **Simple, simple, simple.** Nearly everyone is looking for fast, convenient foods that are simple to prepare. Simplicity also can encompass cost-effectiveness. I accept this set of requirements as a dietary fact of twenty-first-century life, so I hope you will find that these quick and easy smoothie recipes work for you in meeting those goals with flying colors.

We don't have to make elaborate meal preparations to load up on nutrients. Smoothies are meant to be a fun way to mix your favorite superfruits in a format anyone can find convenient, tasty, and packed with maximal nutrient content!

HIGH NUTRIENT CONTENTS FOR ALL SMOOTHIES
Because these recipes use nutrient-enriched superfruits, *fortified* soy milk, *fortified* low-fat or nonfat yogurt, and flaxseeds, the general nutritional quality of the smoothies is multiplied to a level high enough to amply cover most nutrient categories. For this reason, no individual nutrient summary is included with the smoothie recipes.

Brazilian Blast

1 cup low-fat or nonfat vanilla yogurt plus extra for garnish
1 cup mango chunks
1 cup açaí juice
2 strawberries

FAVORITE SUPERFRUIT SUBSTITUTES
- ► Instead of mango, try red guava or papaya.
- ► Add ¼ cup soft tofu for extra protein and texture.

Blend the 1 cup yogurt, mango, and açaí juice until smooth. Pour into two tall glasses and refrigerate for 30 minutes (or freeze for 5 minutes) to thicken. Make a small slit in each strawberry and slide one onto the rim of each glass. Swirl a spoonful of the remaining yogurt on top of each smoothie. Serve with a long spoon and straw.

MAKES 2 servings

Açaí Peanut Fusion

1 cup fortified soy milk
1 cup açaí juice
4 tablespoons smooth or crunchy peanut butter
1 ripe banana
Handful of flaxseeds

Blend all ingredients until smooth. Serve with a long spoon and straw.

MAKES 2 servings

Apple-Mango Custard Smoothie

1 cup apple chunks
½ cup mango chunks
½ cup apple juice

½ cup canned vanilla custard
Handful of flaxseeds, optional
1 tablespoon ground cinnamon
2 sweet cherries on stems

Blend apple, mango, apple juice, custard, and flaxseeds until smooth. Pour into a tall glass, and garnish with cinnamon and cherries. Serve with a long spoon and straw.

MAKES 1 serving

Avocado-Pineapple Smoothie

1 cup avocado chunks
½ cup pineapple chunks
½ cup mango chunks
1 cup pineapple juice
Handful of flaxseeds, optional

Blend all ingredients until smooth. Pour into a tall glass, and serve with a long spoon and straw.

MAKES 1 serving

Banana-Mango PB Smoothie

½ ripe banana
½ cup mango chunks
1 cup fortified vanilla soy milk
2 tablespoons smooth or crunchy peanut butter
2 tablespoons raw peanuts

FAVORITE SUPERFRUIT SUBSTITUTES
▶ Instead of mango, try papaya.
▶ Instead of peanut butter, try other nut butters such as pecan, almond, or hazelnut.

Blend all ingredients until smooth. Pour into a tall glass, and serve with a long spoon and straw.

MAKES 1 serving

Banana-Mango Smoothie

1 ripe banana
1 cup mango chunks
2 cups 100 percent orange juice with pulp
Handful of flaxseeds, optional
1 tablespoon ground nutmeg

Blend banana, mango, orange juice, and flaxseeds. Pour into two tall glasses, and garnish each smoothie with ½ tablespoon nutmeg. Serve with a long spoon and straw.

MAKES 2 servings

Tropical Superfruit Smoothie

1 ripe banana
½ cup mango chunks
½ cup papaya chunks
½ cup pineapple chunks
2 cups 100 percent orange juice with pulp
Handful of flaxseeds, optional
1 tablespoon ground cinnamon
4 sweet cherries on stems

Blend banana, fruit chunks, orange juice, and flaxseeds until smooth. Pour into two tall glasses, and garnish each smoothie with ½ tablespoon cinnamon and two cherries. Serve with a long spoon and straw.

MAKES 2 servings

Blackberry Smoothie

1 cup blackberries
1 cup low-fat or nonfat vanilla yogurt (for extra chill, use frozen yogurt)
3 packets Splenda (or to taste, to offset slight sourness of blackberries) or
⅓ cup pineapple juice
4 cups (1 liter) fortified soy milk
8 sweet cherries on stems

Blend blackberries, yogurt, Splenda, and soy milk until smooth. Pour into tall glasses, and garnish each smoothie with one or two cherries. Serve with a long spoon and straw.

MAKES 5 servings

Blackberry-Grape Smoothie

1 cup fresh or frozen blackberries
2 cups Concord grape juice
½ cup fortified vanilla soy milk
Handful of flaxseeds, optional
½ cup low-fat or nonfat vanilla yogurt

Blend blackberries, grape juice, soy milk, and flaxseeds until smooth. Pour into two tall glasses, and scoop ¼ cup yogurt on top of each smoothie. Serve with a long spoon and straw.

MAKES 2 servings

Blackberry-Melon-Kiwi Smoothie

½ cup blackberries
½ cup cantaloupe chunks
1 kiwifruit, with or without skin (skin provides extra fiber)
1½ cups fortified vanilla soy milk
½ cup low-fat or nonfat vanilla yogurt
1 teaspoon vanilla extract
Handful of flaxseeds, optional

Blend all ingredients until smooth. Pour into two tall glasses, and serve with a long spoon and straw.

MAKES 2 servings

Morning Energy Blueberry Smoothie

1 cup frozen blueberries
2 ripe bananas
2 cups fortified vanilla soy milk
1 cup low-fat or nonfat vanilla yogurt
1 cup fortified whole-grain cereal such as Total or Shreddies

---

FAVORITE SUPERFRUIT SUBSTITUTES
► Instead of blueberries, make mango, strawberries, papaya, or red guava the featured superfruit.
► Add ½ cup soft tofu for extra protein and delicious texture.

Blend blueberries, bananas, soy milk, and yogurt until mixture has a smooth consistency for spooning. (Show kids how to do this for themselves.) Pour into four bowls, and top each with ¼ cup cereal. Serve with a spoon.

MAKES 4 servings

Blueberry-Banana Blast

1 cup low-fat or nonfat vanilla yogurt plus extra for garnish
2 cups 100 percent or blended blueberry juice
2 small ripe bananas
2 strawberries

Blend the 1 cup yogurt with blueberry juice; add bananas and continue to blend until smooth. Pour into two tall glasses and refrigerate for 30 minutes (or freeze for 5 minutes) to thicken. Make a small slit in each strawberry and slide one onto the rim of each glass. Swirl a spoonful of the remaining yogurt on top of each smoothie. Serve with a long spoon and straw.

MAKES 2 servings

Cherryets of Fire

1 cup pitted canned or fresh sweet cherries
½ cup low-fat or nonfat vanilla yogurt
2 cups fortified vanilla soy milk
2 pinches of ground cloves
2 strawberries
1 tablespoon ground cinnamon

Blend cherries, yogurt, soy milk, and cloves until smooth. Pour into two tall glasses. Make a small slit in each strawberry and slide one onto the rim of each glass. Sprinkle ½ tablespoon cinnamon on top of each smoothie. Serve with a long spoon and straw.

MAKES 2 servings

Citrus Tonic

1 small ripe banana
1 cup mandarins
½ cup grapefruit segments
⅓ cup lime segments
2 cups 100 percent orange juice with pulp
½ cup low-fat or nonfat vanilla yogurt
2 lemon slices

Blend all ingredients except lemon until smooth. Pour into two tall glasses. Slit the lemon slices and slide one onto the rim of each glass. Serve with a long spoon and straw.

MAKES 2 servings

Cocktail Mega-Smoothie

½ cup papaya chunks
½ cup mango chunks
½ cup pineapple chunks
½ cup unpeeled Red Delicious apple segments
2 small carrots
2 cups fortified vanilla soy milk
Handful of flaxseeds, optional
4 celery stalks with leaves

Blend all ingredients except celery until smooth. Pour into two tall glasses. Place two celery stalks in each glass; garnish with celery leaves. Serve with a long spoon and straw.

MAKES 2 servings

Cocoberry Smoothie

½ cup blueberries
½ cup red raspberries
½ cup blackberries
2 cups fortified vanilla soy milk
½ cup coconut milk
½ cup low-fat or nonfat vanilla yogurt
Handful of flaxseeds, optional

Blend all ingredients until smooth. Pour into two tall glasses, and serve with a long spoon and straw.

MAKES 2 servings

Cranberry-Banana Smoothie

¼ cup frozen cranberries plus 4 dried cranberries for garnish
1 ripe banana
1 cup fortified soy milk
Handful of flaxseeds

2 packets Splenda
1 lime, sliced thick
2 tablespoons low-fat or nonfat vanilla yogurt

Blend the frozen cranberries, banana, soy milk, flaxseeds, and Splenda until smooth. Pour into a tall glass. Slit one lime slice and slide it onto the rim of the glass. Drop yogurt on top of smoothie, squeeze juice of remaining lime on yogurt, and sprinkle with remaining dried cranberries. Serve with a long spoon and straw.

MAKES 1 serving

Orange-Fig Smoothie

4 black mission figs (remove stems)
1 ripe banana
1 cup 100 percent orange juice with maximum pulp
1 cup low-fat or nonfat vanilla or strawberry yogurt
1 to 2 packets Splenda or ⅓ cup pineapple juice
8 blueberries

Blend all ingredients except blueberries until smooth. Pour into two tall glasses, and sprinkle four blueberries over each smoothie. Serve with a long spoon and straw.

MAKES 2 servings

Grape-Peach Supreme

1 cup Concord grape juice
½ cup canned peaches plus extra for garnish
1 cup fortified vanilla soy milk
1 tablespoon sunflower seeds

FAVORITE SUPERFRUIT SUBSTITUTES
Instead of peach, try mango, papaya, or red guava.

Blend grape juice, the ½ cup peaches, soy milk, and sunflower seeds until smooth. Pour into two tall glasses, and place one of the remaining peach segments on top of each smoothie. Serve with a long spoon and straw.

MAKES 2 servings

Grape-Kiwi Smoothie

½ cup grapes
1 kiwifruit, with or without skin (skin provides extra fiber)
1½ cups fortified vanilla soy milk
½ cup low-fat or nonfat vanilla yogurt
½ tablespoon ground nutmeg

Blend all ingredients except nutmeg until smooth. Pour into two tall glasses, and sprinkle ¼ teaspoon nutmeg over each smoothie. Serve with a long spoon and straw.

MAKES 2 servings

Green Power Smoothie

1 kiwifruit, with or without skin (skin provides extra fiber)
½ cup green ("white") grapes
½ cup avocado chunks
1½ cups fortified vanilla soy milk
½ cup low-fat or nonfat vanilla yogurt
4 celery stalks with leaves

Blend all ingredients except celery until smooth. Pour into two tall glasses, and place two celery stalks in each glass; garnish with celery leaves. Serve with a long spoon and straw.

MAKES 2 servings

Guava-Banana Smoothie

1 ripe red guava, cut into coarse chunks (skin and seeds optional)
1 ripe banana

Handful of flaxseeds

1 cup fortified soy milk

1 lime, half for squeezing juice, half sliced for garnish

2 packets Splenda (or to taste) or ⅓ cup pineapple juice

2 ice cubes

Blend guava, banana, flaxseeds, and soy milk until smooth; squeeze half a lime for its juice, add Splenda, and ice cubes, and blend again until smooth. Pour into two tall glasses. Slit two lime slices and slide one onto the rim of each glass. Serve with a long spoon and straw.

MAKES 2 servings

Kiwi Cooler

1 kiwifruit, with or without skin (skin provides extra fiber)

½ cup green ("white") grapes

¼ cup grated lemon peel

1½ cups sparkling mineral water or zero-calorie ginger ale

2 tablespoons honey

2 cucumber slices

2 lemon slices

2 mint sprigs

Blend kiwifruit, grapes, lemon peel, mineral water, and honey until smooth. Pour into two tall glasses, and garnish each with a cucumber slice, lemon slice, and mint sprig. Serve with a long spoon and straw.

MAKES 2 servings

Strawberry-Kiwi Smoothie

4 strawberries

2 kiwifruits, with or without skin (skin provides extra fiber)

2 cups fortified vanilla soy milk

1 cup low-fat or nonfat vanilla yogurt

4 tablespoons (2 ounces) flaked almonds

Blend all ingredients except almonds until smooth. Pour into two tall glasses, and sprinkle 2 tablespoons almonds over each smoothie. Serve with a long spoon and straw.

MAKES 2 servings

Kiwi-Melon Custard Smoothie

2 kiwifruits—skin optional for extra fiber
1 cup cantaloupe chunks
1 cup fortified vanilla soy milk
¼ cup soft tofu
½ cup canned vanilla custard
Handful of flaxseeds, optional

Blend all ingredients until smooth. Pour into two tall glasses, and serve with a long spoon and straw.

MAKES 2 servings

Mango Vanilla Smoothie

2 medium mangoes, with or without skin, diced
1 cup fortified soy milk
1 cup low-fat or nonfat vanilla yogurt
Handful of flaxseeds
2 tablespoons lemon juice
2 packets Splenda or ⅓ cup pineapple juice
2 tablespoons vanilla extract
10 frozen blueberries

FAVORITE SUPERFRUIT SUBSTITUTES
Instead of mango, try red guava, papaya, pitted cherries, or fresh or frozen blueberries.

Blend all ingredients except blueberries until smooth. Pour into two tall glasses, and stir five blueberries into each glass for colorful garnish and extra nutrients. Serve with a long spoon and straw.

MAKES 2 servings

Mango-Lemonberry Blast

1 cup mango chunks
1 cup low-fat or nonfat vanilla or strawberry yogurt
4 ounces sugar-free liquid lemonade
1 to 2 packets Splenda or ⅓ cup pineapple juice as optional sweetener
5 large strawberries

Blend all ingredients except strawberries until smooth; add strawberries and blend briefly until they begin to break into chunks (about 5 seconds). Pour into two tall glasses, and serve with a long spoon.

MAKES 2 servings

Mangoberry Smoothie

1 cup mango chunks
1 cup low-fat or nonfat vanilla yogurt
1 cup cranberry juice
1 to 2 packets Splenda or ⅓ cup pineapple juice as optional sweetener
6 large red raspberries

Blend all ingredients except raspberries until smooth. Pour into two tall glasses and drop three raspberries onto top of each glass. Serve with a long spoon.

MAKES 2 servings

Superberry Melon Smoothie

1 cup watermelon chunks with seeds (seeds provide extra nutrients
    when blended)
½ cup red raspberries

½ cup blueberries
½ cup red grapes
1 cup 100 percent orange juice with pulp
Handful of flaxseeds, optional

Blend all ingredients until smooth. Pour into two tall glasses, and serve with a long spoon and straw.

MAKES 2 servings

Mango-Orange Smoothie

½ cup mango chunks
½ cup 100 percent orange juice with pulp
1½ cups fortified vanilla soy milk
2 tablespoons honey
Handful of flaxseeds, optional

Blend all ingredients until smooth. Pour into two tall glasses, and serve with a long spoon and straw.

Makes 2 servings

Oriental Smoothie

1 kiwifruit, with or without skin (skin provides extra fiber)
½ cup mango chunks
½ cup apple chunks
½ cup mandarins
1 cup 100 percent orange juice with pulp
Handful of flaxseeds, optional

Blend all ingredients until smooth. Pour into two tall glasses, and serve with a long spoon and straw.

MAKES 2 servings

Papaya-Banana-Lime Smoothie

2 ripe bananas
2 cups peeled and seeded ripe papaya (ripe when aroma is fruity and skin is
    soft), cubed (seeds optional for extra nutrients and tangy taste)
Handful of flaxseeds
2 cups fortified soy milk
2 packets Splenda as optional sweetener
¼ cup pineapple juice
½ lime

Blend bananas, papaya, flaxseeds, and soy milk until smooth; add Splenda
and the ¼ cup pineapple juice, and blend again. Squeeze juice of the lime
into the mixture and stir. Pour into four tall glasses, and serve with a long
spoon and straw.

MAKES 4 servings

Papaya-Pineapple Potion

1 ripe banana
½ Red Delicious apple
½ cup papaya chunks
½ cup pineapple chunks
1 cup 100 percent orange juice with pulp
Handful of flaxseeds, optional

Blend all ingredients until smooth. Pour into two tall glasses, and serve
with a long spoon and straw.

MAKES 2 servings

Tangy Papaya Smoothie

½ cup papaya chunks
½ cup pink grapefruit segments
1½ cups cranberry juice

2 red raspberries
½ lime, sliced into 2 sections

Blend papaya, grapefruit, and cranberry juice until smooth. Pour into two tall glasses. Drop a raspberry into each smoothie; slit lime sections and slide one onto the rim of each glass. Serve with a long spoon and straw.

MAKES 2 servings

Pomelon Smoothie

½ cup pomegranate seeds plus extra for garnish
1 cup watermelon (with seeds for extra nutrients!)
1½ cups fortified vanilla soy milk

Blend the ½ cup pomegranate seeds, watermelon, and soy milk until smooth. Pour into two tall glasses, and garnish top of each smoothie with remaining pomegranate seeds. Serve with a long spoon and straw.

MAKES 2 servings

Pom Peach Smoothie

1 cup canned peach halves
½ cup pomegranate seeds plus extra seeds for garnish
1 cup 100 percent orange juice with pulp
½ cup low-fat or nonfat vanilla yogurt

Blend peaches, the ½ cup pomegranate seeds, and orange juice until smooth. Pour into two tall glasses, and garnish with remaining pomegranate seeds. Serve with a long spoon and straw.

MAKES 2 servings

Raspberry Vanilla Swirl

1 cup red raspberries plus 4 berries for garnish
1 cup fortified vanilla soy milk

½ cup low-fat or nonfat vanilla yogurt plus extra for garnish
1 teaspoon vanilla extract

Blend the 1 cup raspberries, soy milk, the ½ cup yogurt, and vanilla until smooth. Pour into two tall glasses. Swirl a spoonful of the remaining yogurt on top of each smoothie to decorate, and add two raspberries to each glass. Serve with a long spoon and straw.

MAKES 2 servings

Scarlet Berry Power

1 cup red raspberries plus 4 berries for garnish
½ cup blueberries
½ cup strawberries
½ cup dark grapes
1½ cups fortified vanilla soy milk
½ cup low-fat or nonfat vanilla yogurt plus extra for garnish
Handful of flaxseeds, optional

Blend the 1 cup raspberries, blueberries, strawberries, grapes, soy milk, the ½ cup yogurt, and flaxseeds until smooth. Pour into two tall glasses. Swirl a spoonful of the remaining yogurt on top, and add two raspberries to each glass to decorate. Serve with a long spoon and straw.

MAKES 2 servings

Strawberry-Raspberry Vanilla Smoothie

¾ cup strawberries
1 cup fortified soy milk
½ cup low-fat or nonfat vanilla yogurt
1 teaspoon vanilla extract
4 fresh or frozen red raspberries

Blend all ingredients except raspberries until smooth. Pour into two tall glasses, and add two raspberries to each glass. Serve each smoothie with one white and one red straw and a long spoon.

MAKES 2 servings

Strawberry Cran Smoothie

1 ripe banana
1 cup strawberries plus 2 sliced berries for garnish
½ cup cranberry juice
½ cup fortified soy milk
½ cup low-fat or nonfat vanilla yogurt

Blend banana, the 1 cup strawberries, cranberry juice, soy milk, and yogurt until smooth. Pour into two tall glasses, and divide the sliced strawberries between the glasses. Serve with a long spoon and straw.

MAKES 2 servings

Garden of Eden Smoothie

One of the most talked-about dietary plans is the Garden of Eden concept (also called the "Portfolio" diet), which combines all the foods shown in scientific studies to lower levels of blood cholesterol. Key ingredients are soy products (fortified soy milk, tofu), phytosterol sources (banana, flaxseeds, strawberry seeds), prebiotic fiber (oatmeal, barley, psyllium, tofu, strawberries, banana), and nuts (almonds).

1 ripe banana
1 cup fresh strawberries plus 2 sliced berries for garnish
1 cup fortified soy milk
½ cup smooth tofu
½ cup low-fat or nonfat vanilla yogurt
¼ cup ground flaxseeds
8 almonds

Blend banana, the 1 cup strawberries, soy milk, tofu, yogurt, and flaxseeds until smooth. Pour into two tall glasses, and divide the sliced strawberries and almonds between the glasses. Serve with a long spoon and straw.

MAKES 2 servings

Breakfast Ideas and Snacks

I'm a fan of regularly using instant hot oatmeal or Cream of Wheat to start my day and for afternoon or evening snacks. Each takes less than two minutes to prepare in the microwave, has among the best glycemic load and appetite-dampening effects known among foods, and is an easy high-fiber solution that invites a superfruit companion or two.

Keep in mind the FDA-approved health claim allowed for prebiotic fiber in products containing whole oats, barley, psyllium, or wheat. When used regularly over weeks, getting just 0.75 gram (750 milligrams) per serving of prebiotic fiber can reduce blood cholesterol levels and yield numerous potential benefits against cardiovascular diseases and some types of cancer.

Now pair the oatmeal with a serving or two of high-fiber, high-nutrient superfruits plus some *pro*biotic benefit from yogurt, and you are really in business for giving your body satisfying, high-impact nutrition. Fiber may be the most important nutrient for maintaining the health benefits and lowered disease risk that superfruits naturally offer. Many of the recipes in this section can give you ideas for fulfilling your fiber quota (30 or more grams per day) while making a delicious and healthy start to your morning!

Smooth Superfruit Oatmeal

½ cup oatmeal flakes (instant oatmeal)
⅓ cup fresh or frozen blueberries
2 tablespoons ground cinnamon (optional)
⅓ cup low-fat or nonfat vanilla yogurt
Handful of walnuts or pumpkin seeds

Place oatmeal in a microwavable bowl, and add about 2 ounces of water (adjust to suit your preference for texture). Microwave on high for about 80 seconds. Add blueberries first (if they are frozen, work them into the hot oatmeal to melt), sprinkle the cinnamon if desired, and then pour the yogurt. Top with nuts and serve.

MAKES 1 serving

SUPERFRUIT RECIPE SNAPSHOT: BLUEBERRIES
High Nutrient Content: prebiotic fiber, dietary minerals
High Phytochemical Content: polyphenols (anthocyanins, proanthocyanidins, resveratrol)
Color Code: blue

Superfruit Starter Medley

1 cup mango chunks
6 black mission figs
4 pitted dates
1 kiwifruit, sliced (skin optional for extra dietary fiber)
20 blueberries
2 small bunches of red grapes

Arrange all fruits evenly on two plates and serve.

MAKES 2 servings

SUPERFRUIT RECIPE SNAPSHOT: MANGO, FIGS, DATES, KIWIFRUIT, BLUEBERRIES, RED GRAPES

High Nutrient Content: prebiotic fiber, antioxidant A-C-E vitamins, B vitamins, dietary minerals

High Phytochemical Content: carotenoids (alpha- and beta-carotene, beta-cryptoxanthin, lutein, violaxanthin); polyphenols (mixed flavonoids—anthocyanins, quercetin, gallic acid, gallotannins, rhamnetin, cyanidin and xanthone glycosides, chlorophyll, resveratrol)

Color Code: orange-yellow, red-tan, green, blue-purple

Superfruit Pita

½ ripe banana, crushed

2 pitted dates, diced

1 tablespoon dried blackcurrants

1 6-inch whole-grain pita

2 tablespoons smooth or crunchy peanut butter

2 strawberries, thinly sliced

In a small bowl, combine banana, dates, and currants. Toast pita or microwave for a few seconds; cut open. Spread peanut butter inside pita, stuff with banana mixture, and top with strawberries. Eat while still warm or reheat.

MAKES 1 serving

SUPERFRUIT RECIPE SNAPSHOT: DATES, BLACKCURRANTS, STRAWBERRIES

High Nutrient Content: antioxidant A-C-E vitamins, B vitamins, dietary minerals

High Phytochemical Content: carotenoids (beta-carotene); polyphenols (anthocyanins, particularly pelargonidin, and ellagic acid and ellagitannins in the strawberry achenes, delphinidin and cyanidin glycosides and rutinosides, quercetin, hydroxycinnamic acids, proanthocyanidins)

Color Code: red-tan, black

Superfruit Applesauce

2 cups applesauce
4 dates, quartered
¼ cup raisins
¼ cup dried cranberries
¼ cup goji berries (wolfberries)
¼ cup shredded coconut
¼ cup almond slivers
2 tablespoons ground cinnamon

FAVORITE SUPERFRUIT SUBSTITUTES
For any of the superfruits listed, try fig slices, red grapes, dried or fresh blueberries, red raspberries, dried blackcurrants, dried cranberries, date slices, or walnut pieces.

Mix applesauce, dates, raisins, cranberries, and goji berries in a microwavable bowl. Microwave on high for about 90 seconds. Spoon into serving bowls, garnish with equal amounts of coconut and almonds, and sprinkle cinnamon evenly. Serve warm.

MAKES 2 to 4 servings

SUPERFRUIT RECIPE SNAPSHOT: DATES, RAISINS, CRANBERRIES, GOJI BERRIES (WOLFBERRIES)
High Nutrient Content: prebiotic fiber, antioxidant A-C-E vitamins, B vitamins, dietary minerals
High Phytochemical Content: carotenoids (beta-carotene, zeaxanthin, beta-cryptoxanthin, lycopene); polyphenols (anthocyanins, oligomeric proanthocyanidins, other mixed polyphenols such as tannins, quercetin, apigenin, ellagic acid)
Color Code: red-tan, blue-purple

Superfruit-Stuffed Cantaloupe

2 large cantaloupes, halved and seeded
1 small orange, sectioned
1 unpeeled Red Delicious apple, cubed
2 black mission figs, sliced into small strips
1 cup fresh blueberries
½ cup fresh strawberries, sliced
1 cup low-fat or nonfat vanilla yogurt
2 tablespoons ground cinnamon

With a melon baller or small spoon, scoop out 2 to 3 cups of cantaloupe balls and place in a large bowl; leave enough cantaloupe in the shells to be eaten separately. Add orange, apple, figs, blueberries, and strawberries to canteloupe in bowl, and stir to combine. Place each cantaloupe shell in a serving bowl. Divide fruit mixture evenly among the four shells. Spoon ¼ cup yogurt onto each serving, and sprinkle with cinnamon. Serve for breakfast or brunch with whole-grain, low-fat muffins.

MAKES 4 servings

SUPERFRUIT RECIPE SNAPSHOT: ORANGE, FIGS, BLUEBERRIES, STRAWBERRIES
High Nutrient Content: antioxidant A-C-E vitamins, B vitamins, dietary minerals
High Phytochemical Content: carotenoids (beta-cryptoxanthin, beta-carotene); polyphenols (hesperidin, anthocyanins, proanthocyanidins, ellagic acid, resveratrol)
Color Code: orange, red-tan, black, blue

Superfruit Starter Compote

3 large unpeeled Red Delicious apples, cut into thick chunks
½ cup pitted dried plums (prunes)
¾ cup dried blackcurrants
½ cup dried cranberries

1 orange, peeled and cut into 8 pieces (with pith)

⅓ cup grated orange peel

4 packets Splenda

2 tablespoons ground cinnamon

2 tablespoons cornstarch

½ cup walnut pieces

In a saucepan, combine apples, plums, currants, cranberries, and orange pieces; add 3 cups of water. Heat on medium and stir occasionally until hot; reduce heat to low and simmer for 10 minutes. Stir in orange peel, Splenda, and cinnamon. In a small bowl, combine cornstarch with 3 tablespoons of water; stir into saucepan. Raise heat to medium and cook, stirring constantly, until sauce thickens. Serve hot or cold topped with cinnamon and walnuts on yogurt, whole-grain cereal, or baked items.

MAKES 4 servings

SUPERFRUIT RECIPE SNAPSHOT: DRIED PLUMS (PRUNES), BLACKCURRANTS, CRANBERRIES, ORANGE

High Nutrient Content: protein, prebiotic fiber, antioxidant A-C-E vitamins (diminished by heating), B vitamins, dietary minerals

High Phytochemical Content: carotenoids (beta-cryptoxanthin, beta-carotene); polyphenols (anthocyanins, particularly delphinidin and cyanidin glycosides and rutinosides, catechins, proanthocyanidins, chlorogenic acid, quercetin, hydroxycinnamic acid)

Color Code: purple-black, red-tan, orange

Whole-Oat Berry Scones

3 tablespoons canola oil

2 cups whole-oat flour

4 packets Splenda

2 tablespoons baking powder

½ cup fortified soy milk

¾ cup low-fat or nonfat vanilla yogurt

½ cup dried blackcurrants

⅓ cup dried goji berries (wolfberries)

¼ cup 100 percent orange juice with pulp

Preheat oven to 400°F. Coat an 8-inch cake pan with canola oil. Combine remaining ingredients in a large bowl and stir until well blended. Pour into the pan and bake 18 to 25 minutes, until top is golden brown and a knife inserted in center comes out clean. Serve hot, or cool for 20 minutes. Cut into scone wedges and serve alone, in a bowl with yogurt, or with your favorite superfruit jam.

MAKES 4 to 6 servings

SUPERFRUIT RECIPE SNAPSHOT: BLACKCURRANTS, GOJI BERRIES (WOLFBERRIES)

High Nutrient Content: prebiotic fiber, dietary minerals

High Phytochemical Content: carotenoids (zeaxanthin, beta-cryptoxanthin, beta-carotene, lycopene); polyphenols (anthocyanins, particularly delphinidin and cyanidin glycosides and rutinosides, quercetin, hydroxycinnamic acids, proanthocyanidins, ellagic acid)

Color Code: black, red-tan

Poached Papaya

1 medium papaya, halved and cored

About 2 cups 100 percent orange juice with pulp

2 tablespoons ground cinnamon

2 scoops low-fat vanilla frozen yogurt

½ cup triple-fruit (orange-grapefruit-lemon) marmalade

FAVORITE SUPERFRUIT SUBSTITUTES

► Instead of papaya, try red guava, orange, or mango as the main superfruit—reduce cooking times accordingly.

► Instead of marmalade, try fig slices, dried or fresh blueberries, dried blackcurrants, dried cranberries, or date slices.

Place papaya halves, cut-side up, in a stove-top pan. Add enough orange juice to cover papaya, and sprinkle with cinnamon. Place on medium heat. Cover pan, reduce heat to low, and simmer 10 to 15 minutes, until papaya is tender. Remove pan from heat, allow to cool, and refrigerate until chilled. Transfer to two bowls or plates, and place one scoop of frozen yogurt per serving plus ¼ cup marmalade onto each papaya half. Serve with whole wheat breadsticks or Indian bread called naan.

MAKES 2 servings

SUPERFRUIT RECIPE SNAPSHOT: PAPAYA
High Nutrient Content: antioxidant A-C-E vitamins
High Phytochemical Content: carotenoids (beta-cryptoxanthin, beta-carotene, lycopene); polyphenols (anthocyanins, tannins)
Color Code: orange-yellow

Premium Fast-Break Dried Superfruit Medley

2 dried mango slices, diced
¼ cup dried blueberries
¼ cup dried cranberries
¼ cup goji berries (wolfberries)
¼ cup walnut pieces or unsalted roasted almonds
¼ cup Cheerios or any firm, high-nutrient, whole-grain cereal—check the Nutrition Facts panel!

Combine all ingredients in a ziplock bag and go!

MAKES 1 serving

SUPERFRUIT RECIPE SNAPSHOT: MANGO, BLUEBERRIES, CRANBERRIES, GOJI BERRIES (WOLFBERRIES)

High Nutrient Content: prebiotic fiber, antioxidant A-C-E vitamins, dietary minerals

High Phytochemical Content: carotenoids (alpha- and beta-carotene, beta-cryptoxanthin, lutein, violaxanthin, zeaxanthin, lycopene); polyphenols (quercetin, gallic acid, gallotannins, rhamnetin, cyanidin and xanthone glycosides, proanthocyanidins, resveratrol)

Color Code: yellow, blue, red-tan

Basic Fast-Break Dried Superfruit Medley

2 pitted dates, diced

¼ cup raisins

¼ cup dried blackcurrants

2 black mission figs, sliced

¼ cup unsalted roasted sunflower or pumpkin seeds

¼ cup Cheerios or other firm, high-nutrient, whole-grain cereal

Combine all ingredients in a ziplock bag and go!

MAKES 1 serving

SUPERFRUIT RECIPE SNAPSHOT: DATES, RAISINS, BLACKCURRANTS, FIGS

High Nutrient Content: prebiotic fiber, antioxidant A-C-E vitamins, B vitamins, dietary minerals

High Phytochemical Content: carotenoids (beta-carotene); polyphenols (anthocyanins, particularly delphinidin and cyanidin glycosides and rutinosides, quercetin, hydroxycinnamic acids, proanthocyanidins);

Color Code: purple-black

Fancy Superfruit Yogurt Parfait

1 cup low-fat or nonfat vanilla yogurt

1 cup mandarin orange segments

¼ cup confectioners' sugar (powdered sugar)

1 large banana, cut into small pieces

1 cup strawberries, sliced

½ cup blueberries

1 cup mango chunks

½ cup pineapple chunks

¼ cup shredded coconut

Spoon ¼ cup yogurt into each of four tall parfait glasses or glass dishes. Layer oranges evenly over the yogurt, and sprinkle servings with a third of the confectioners' sugar. Layer banana slices on top, and sprinkle with another third of the confectioners' sugar. Combine strawberries, blueberries, mango, and pineapple chunks; spoon mixture onto each serving, and sprinkle remaining third of the confectioners' sugar on top. Garnish with coconut and serve.

MAKES 4 servings

SUPERFRUIT RECIPE SNAPSHOT: ORANGES, STRAWBERRIES, BLUEBERRIES, MANGO

High Nutrient Content: prebiotic fiber, antioxidant A-C-E vitamins, B vitamins, dietary minerals

High Phytochemical Content: carotenoids (alpha- and beta-carotene, beta-cryptoxanthin, lutein, violaxanthin); polyphenols (hesperidin, anthocyanins, quercetin, gallic acid, gallotannins, rhamnetin, cyanidin and xanthone glycosides, proanthocyanidins, resveratrol, ellagic acid, ellagitannins)

Color Code: orange-yellow, red, blue

Salads

Salads are a no-fail format for enriching your diet with delectable tastes, textures, and nutrients. And talk about making green leafy salads more interesting, even for kids? Load each serving with pieces of superfruits—and watch the attitudes change for the better!

Avocado Superfruit Salad

4 plates or bowls with crisp salad greens spread evenly
1 ripe avocado, peeled and cut into wedges
1 navel orange, sectioned
1 medium unpeeled ripe mango, cut into chunks (peel optional; include for additional dietary fiber)
½ cup mixed dried cranberries and dried blackcurrants
8 cherry tomatoes
⅓ cup walnut pieces
Unsaturated-fat salad dressing, olive oil, or canola oil

Arrange greens in four salad plates or bowls. Combine remaining ingredients except the dressing in a bowl; divide the mixture among the four plates. Top with dressing and serve.

MAKES 4 servings

SUPERFRUIT RECIPE SNAPSHOT: ORANGE, MANGO, CRANBERRIES, BLACKCURRANTS
High Nutrient Content: prebiotic fiber, antioxidant A-C-E vitamins, B vitamins, dietary minerals, phytosterols, omega fats
High Phytochemical Content: carotenoids (alpha- and beta-carotene, beta-cryptoxanthin, lutein, violaxanthin); polyphenols (hesperidin, anthocyanins, quercetin, gallic acid, gallotannins, rhamnetin, cyanidin and xanthone glycosides, proanthocyanidins, resveratrol, ellagic acid, ellagitannins)
Color Code: orange-yellow, green, red-tan, purple-black

Mango Black-Bean Salad

1 ripe mango, diced (peel optional; include for additional dietary fiber)
1 can (16–17 ounces, 500 ml) baked black beans, rinsed and drained
¼ yellow sweet pepper, diced
¼ red sweet pepper, diced
1 can (16–17 ounces, 500 ml) whole-kernel corn ("peaches and cream")
2 small onions, diced
¼ cup coriander, chopped
½ cup walnut pieces
½ cup low-calorie barbecue sauce
8 curved romaine leaves
1 lime, cut into 8 sections

In a bowl, stir together mango, beans, peppers, corn, onions, coriander, walnuts, and sauce. Spoon ⅔ cup of the mixture into each lettuce leaf, add a lime section, and serve.

MAKES 8 servings

SUPERFRUIT RECIPE SNAPSHOT: MANGO (WITH BLACK BEANS AND CAROTENOID-RICH ROMAINE, PEPPERS, AND CORN)
High Nutrient Content: protein, prebiotic fiber, antioxidant A-C-E vitamins, dietary minerals, phytosterols, omega fats
High Phytochemical Content: carotenoids (alpha- and beta-carotene, beta-cryptoxanthin, lutein, violaxanthin); polyphenols (quercetin, gallic acid, gallotannins, rhamnetin, cyanidin and xanthone glycosides, including mangiferin, especially in mango peel)
Color Code: orange-yellow, black, red, green

Mango Hot Broccoli with Pomegranate Seeds

2 cups broccoli florets
2 tablespoons canola oil
1 tablespoon curry powder

2 tablespoons lemon juice
2 cups mango chunks
About 50 pomegranate seeds, arils intact

Preheat oven to 350°F. Place broccoli in a casserole dish, and pour canola oil, curry powder, and lemon juice evenly over florets. Cover and bake until tender, about 20 minutes. Mix mango chunks into broccoli. Spoon contents onto two salad plates, and sprinkle half of the pomegranate seeds evenly over each plate. Serve warm.

MAKES 2 servings

SUPERFRUIT RECIPE SNAPSHOT: MANGO, POMEGRANATE (WITH NUTRIENT- AND PHYTOCHEMICAL-ENRICHED BROCCOLI)
High Nutrient Content: prebiotic fiber, antioxidant A-C-E vitamins, B vitamins, dietary minerals
High Phytochemical Content: carotenoids (alpha- and beta-carotene, beta-cryptoxanthin, lutein, violaxanthin); polyphenols (quercetin, gallic acid, gallotannins, rhamnetin, cyanidin and xanthone glycosides, punicalagins, mixed anthocyanins)
Color Code: orange-yellow, red, green

Fresh Mega-Superfruit Salad

3 tablespoons lemonade
3 tablespoons liquid honey
3 tablespoons canola oil
1 red grapefruit, sectioned
1 navel orange, sectioned
½ cantaloupe, cut into chunks
½ mango, cut into chunks
1 cup strawberries, chopped
1 cup red grapes
½ cup blueberries

½ cup dried cranberries
¼ cup unsalted, roasted sunflower seeds
4 parsley sprigs

For the dressing, combine lemonade, honey, and canola oil in a mixing cup. Combine all eight fruits in a large bowl. Pour dressing and sprinkle sunflower seeds over fruit, toss, garnish with parsley, and serve.

MAKES 2 to 4 servings

SUPERFRUIT RECIPE SNAPSHOT: ORANGE, MANGO, BLUEBERRIES, CRANBERRIES, STRAWBERRIES, RED GRAPES

High Nutrient Content: prebiotic fiber, antioxidant A-C-E vitamins, B vitamins, dietary minerals

High Phytochemical Content: carotenoids (alpha- and beta-carotene, beta-cryptoxanthin, lutein, violaxanthin); polyphenols (hesperidin, anthocyanins—cyanidin and xanthone glycosides, quercetin, gallic acid, gallotannins, rhamnetin, proanthocyanidins, resveratrol, ellagic acid, ellagitannins)

Color Code: orange-yellow, blue-purple, red

Super Grapefruit Bowls

2 pink grapefruit, halved (seeds included for extra nutrients!)
½ cup unpeeled mango chunks (peel optional; include for additional dietary fiber)
1 navel orange, sectioned
4 tan Turkish figs, dried and sliced
4 strawberries, halved
⅓ cup brown sugar
⅓ cup grated and diced orange peel
1 teaspoon ground cinnamon
4 sweet cherries

With a knife, separate fruit from rind of each grapefruit half, cut into eight spoon-size pieces, and return to rind. Combine mango, orange, figs, and strawberries; spoon mixture into grapefruit rinds. In a small bowl, mix brown sugar, orange peel, and cinnamon; sprinkle over fruits. Place the grapefruit halves in a baking pan and broil 5 to 10 minutes, until juices are bubbling and brown sugar starts to caramelize. Garnish each with a cherry and serve immediately.

MAKES 4 servings

SUPERFRUIT RECIPE SNAPSHOT: MANGO, ORANGE, FIGS, STRAWBERRIES, CHERRIES

High Nutrient Content: prebiotic fiber, antioxidant A-C-E vitamins, B vitamins, dietary minerals

High Phytochemical Content: carotenoids (alpha- and beta-carotene, beta-cryptoxanthin, lutein, violaxanthin); polyphenols (hesperidin, anthocyanins—cyanidin and xanthone glycosides, quercetin, gallic acid, gallotannins, rhamnetin, proanthocyanidins, resveratrol, ellagic acid, ellagitannins)

Color Code: orange-yellow, red-tan

Color Code Fusion Vinaigrette

2 cups fresh spinach
1 small zucchini or cucumber, sliced
1 medium carrot, diced
½ cup cauliflowerets
½ cup mandarin orange segments
4 black mission figs, sliced
½ cup raisins
⅓ cup unsalted roasted pumpkin seeds
⅓ cup canola oil and vinegar dressing

Arrange spinach leaves equally on two plates. Combine remaining ingredients in a bowl; mix well. Scoop salad evenly onto each plate and serve.

MAKES 2 servings

SUPERFRUIT RECIPE SNAPSHOT: ORANGES, FIGS, RAISINS (WITH NUTRIENT- AND PHYTOCHEMICAL-ENRICHED SPINACH, ZUCCHINI, AND CAULIFLOWER)

High Nutrient Content: prebiotic fiber, antioxidant A-C-E vitamins, B vitamins, dietary minerals

High Phytochemical Content: carotenoids (alpha- and beta-carotene, beta-cryptoxanthin, lutein, violaxanthin); polyphenols (hesperidin, anthocyanins—cyanidin and xanthone glycosides, quercetin, gallic acid, gallotannins, rhamnetin, proanthocyanidins, resveratrol)

Color Code: orange-yellow, purple, red-tan, green

Superfruit Waldorf Salad

½ cup diced Red Delicious apple plus apple slices for garnish

½ cup diced celery

⅓ cup red grapes, halved

⅓ cup blueberries

2 tablespoons walnuts, chopped

1 cup bite-size romaine or spinach pieces

¼ cup mayonnaise or low-calorie, polyunsaturated-fat salad dressing

4 parsley sprigs

6 red raspberries

Place diced apple, celery, grapes, blueberries, walnuts, romaine, and mayonnaise in a bowl; toss to combine. Divide salad between two plates or bowls. Garnish each with apple slices, two parsley sprigs, and three raspberries, and serve.

MAKES 2 servings

Sauces

Superfruits offer the sauce chef some amazing combinations of sweet and sour tastes, colors, and nutrient content. Give some thought to how you can best use these advantages in your preparations of sauces for salads, meats, desserts, breakfast toppings, and fruit accents for pouring on colorful vegetable side dishes to tempt the kids!

Superfruit Compote

½ cup brown sugar
¼ cup olive or canola oil
1 tablespoon ground ginger
1 tablespoon curry powder
1 cup unpeeled mango chunks
1 cup canned peach halves, drained
1 cup pineapple chunks, drained
1 cup black mission figs
½ cup pomegranate seeds
½ cup walnut pieces
1 cup fresh or frozen blackberries

Preheat oven to 350°F. In a saucepan, combine brown sugar, oil, ginger, and curry powder; heat on low until dissolved into a syruplike consistency. Arrange mango, peaches, pineapple, and figs in a large baking dish, and coat fruits with syrup. Bake until contents become golden brown, about 40 minutes, basting the fruit occasionally with the syrup. Spoon into dessert dishes alone or with frozen vanilla yogurt. Sprinkle with pomegranate seeds, walnut pieces, and blackberries, and serve.

MAKES 6 to 8 servings

SUPERFRUIT RECIPE SNAPSHOT: MANGO, FIGS, POMEGRANATE, BLACKBERRIES

High Nutrient Content: prebiotic fiber, antioxidant A-C-E vitamins, B vitamins, dietary minerals

High Phytochemical Content: carotenoids (alpha- and beta-carotene, beta-cryptoxanthin, lutein, violaxanthin); polyphenols (anthocyanins—cyanidin and xanthone glycosides, quercetin, gallic acid, gallotannins, rhamnetin, proanthocyanidins, resveratrol, ellagic acid, punicalagins—ellagitannins)

Color Code: orange-yellow, red-tan, black

Superfruit Marmalade Berry Sauce

3 packets Splenda, or ¼ cup pineapple juice

1 tablespoon flour

¾ teaspoon cornstarch

1 cup hot water

½ cup 100 percent orange juice with pulp

⅓ cup grated orange peel

¼ cup orange peel, sliced

3 tablespoons lemon juice

¼ cup lemon peel, sliced

⅓ cup mixed raisins, dried blackcurrants, and diced dried cranberries

1 tablespoon canola oil

Mix Splenda, flour, and cornstarch in a saucepan; stir in 1 cup hot water, and simmer until sauce develops. Add the orange and lemon juices and peels, and stir to combine. Add the raisin-berry mixture and canola oil; stir. Remove from heat and transfer contents to a serving container. Serve hot or cold on yogurt, baked items, or pancakes.

MAKES 2 servings

SUPERFRUIT RECIPE SNAPSHOT: ORANGE, RAISINS, BLACKCURRANTS, CRANBERRIES

High Nutrient Content: antioxidant A-C-E vitamins, B vitamins, dietary minerals

High Phytochemical Content: carotenoids (beta-carotene, beta-cryptoxanthin); polyphenols (hesperidin, anthocyanins—cyanidin and xanthone glycosides, quercetin, gallic acid, gallotannins, rhamnetin, proanthocyanidins, resveratrol, ellagic acid, ellagitannins)

Color Code: orange, blue-black, red-tan

Superfruit Pesto Sauce for Pastas

1 box (about 375 grams) whole-grain pasta, such as penne
½ cup tomato pesto
½ cup papaya, diced
¼ cup dried cranberries
3 tablespoons chopped basil
⅓ cup grated Parmesan cheese

Prepare pasta by boiling until al dente; drain. Combine pasta, pesto, papaya, and cranberries. Divide among four pasta bowls. Sprinkle with basil and grated cheese, and serve.

MAKES 4 servings

Superfruit Hot Chicken Chutney (or for any meat dish)

1 tablespoon canola oil

4 skinless, boneless chicken breast halves

2 sweet onions, diced

½ can (about 4 ounces) cranberry sauce

⅓ cup mango, diced (peel optional; include for additional dietary fiber)

⅓ cup dried cranberries

2 tablespoons red wine vinegar

½ tablespoon dried thyme

Heat canola oil in a large frying pan on medium, add chicken, and cook only until golden, about 4 minutes per side. Transfer chicken to a platter. Add onion to pan, and cook on medium until light brown. Add cranberry sauce, mango, cranberries, vinegar, and thyme, and stir for a few minutes until sauce forms. Return chicken to pan, cover, reduce heat to medium-low, and cook until chicken is completely done (approximately 10 minutes). Serve with your choice of vegetables and whole-grain rice.

MAKES 4 servings

Spiced Superfruit Sauce

1 cup frozen cranberries

1 cup frozen blueberries

1 cup dried blackcurrants

1 cup dried goji berries (wolfberries)

5 cloves

5 allspice sticks

2 cinnamon sticks

2 blades nutmeg

3 cups granulated sugar

Place cranberries, blueberries, currants, and goji berries in a saucepan, and cover with water. Wrap cloves, allspice, cinnamon, and nutmeg in a cheesecloth or similar durable porous bag, and add to pan. Cook on medium for 5 to 10 minutes until cranberries split. Remove spice bag and discard. Add sugar to pan and simmer, stirring, until mixture thickens and forms a sauce. Serve 2 to 3 spoonfuls per serving immediately on baked items or yogurt, or store in the fridge and use as a jam.

MAKES 8 servings

SUPERFRUIT RECIPE SNAPSHOT: CRANBERRIES, BLUEBERRIES, BLACKCURRANTS, GOJI BERRIES (WOLFBERRIES)

High Nutrient Content: prebiotic fiber, antioxidant A-C-E vitamins, B vitamins, dietary minerals

High Phytochemical Content: carotenoids (zeaxanthin, beta-cryptoxanthin, beta-carotene, lycopene); polyphenols (anthocyanins, particularly delphinidin and cyanidin glycosides and rutinosides, quercetin, hydroxycinnamic acids, proanthocyanidins, resveratrol)

Color Code: red-tan, blue-black

Seafood Entrees

Maybe the French were encouraging us with their seafood nickname, *fruits de mar* ("fruits of the sea" or seafood)—superfruits are splendid with fish and other seafoods. There's something magical about how delicate sea tastes and aromas are accented by the presence of fresh fruit. Explore for your favorites, knowing that the Mediterranean diet is at work when you combine a fish dinner with fruit garnishes or side dishes.

Smoked Salmon with Superfruits

4 cups spinach or romaine
1 pound smoked salmon, cut into thin strips
½ tablespoon Dijon mustard
1 tablespoon liquid honey
2 tablespoons lime juice
2 tablespoons grated lime peel
¼ cup canola or olive oil
½ cup chopped mango
½ green or gold kiwifruit, thinly sliced (skin optional for extra dietary fiber)
1 small red onion, thinly sliced
4 tablespoons coarsely chopped coriander

Line four plates with spinach leaves, and top each with ¼ pound salmon. In a small bowl, combine mustard, honey, lime juice, lime peel, and canola oil. Drizzle dressing over salmon.

Spoon equal portions of mango over each plate, followed by a layer of kiwifruit and onion slices. Sprinkle with coriander and serve.

MAKES 4 servings

SUPERFRUIT RECIPE SNAPSHOT: MANGO, KIWIFRUIT (WITH NUTRIENT- AND PHYTOCHEMICAL-ENRICHED SPINACH OR ROMAINE)

High Nutrient Content: protein, antioxidant A-C-E vitamins, B vitamins, dietary minerals, omega fats

High Phytochemical Content: carotenoids (alpha- and beta-carotene, beta-cryptoxanthin, lutein, violaxanthin); polyphenols (mixed flavonoids, quercetin, gallic acid, gallotannins, rhamnetin, cyanidin and xanthone glycosides); chlorophyll

Color Code: green, orange-gold

Salmon with Superfruit Salsa

4 ¼-pound salmon fillets
¼ cup lemon juice
½ tablespoon grated lemon peel
1 tablespoon chopped rosemary
1 lemon, sliced
¼ cup diced pineapple
¼ cup minced onion
3 garlic cloves, minced
2 small jalapeño peppers, diced
1 tomato, diced
½ cup pineapple juice
¼ cup diced red bell pepper
¼ cup diced mango
¼ cup mandarins, diced
8 parsley sprigs

Preheat oven to 350°F. Arrange salmon in a shallow baking dish. Coat fillets with lemon juice and peel, season with rosemary, and top with half of the lemon slices.

Pour ⅓ cup water into the dish. Bake 10 to 20 minutes, until fish flakes easily with a fork. In a medium bowl, mix pineapple, onion, garlic, jalapeño, tomato, pineapple juice, bell pepper, mango, and mandarin. Top baked fillets with fruit salsa, garnish with remaining lemon slices and two parsley sprigs each, and serve.

MAKES 4 servings

SUPERFRUIT RECIPE SNAPSHOT: MANGO, ORANGES (WITH SALMON HIGH IN PROTEIN, OMEGA-3 FATS, AND CAROTENOIDS)
High Nutrient Content: protein, antioxidant A-C-E vitamins, B vitamins, dietary minerals, omega fats
High Phytochemical Content: carotenoids (alpha- and beta-carotene, beta-cryptoxanthin, lutein, violaxanthin); polyphenols (quercetin, gallic acid, gallotannins, rhamnetin, cyanidin and xanthone glycosides, hesperidin)
Color Code: orange-yellow

Mango-Pear Salmon Salad

1 7-ounce can (213 grams) wild Pacific salmon—pink (highest in oil and omega-3 fat), coho (medium color and oil content), or sockeye (reddest, highest in carotenoids but lowest in omega-3 fats)
1 celery stalk, chopped fine
½ cup unsalted sunflower seeds
½ tablespoon curry powder
½ tablespoon mayonnaise
4 large spinach leaves
½ cucumber, sliced
1 14-ounce can (420 grams) Bartlett pear halves, drained
1 cup mango chunks

Drain salmon, place in a bowl, and crush and mix contents with a fork. Add celery, sunflower seeds, curry powder, and mayonnaise; blend well into fish. Arrange spinach leaves on a large plate to cover, and mound cucumber slices in the middle. Alternate pear halves, flat-side up, and spoonfuls of mango chunks in a circle around the cucumber slices. Scoop equal portions of salmon mix into cavity of each pear half. Each serving should contain one to two pear halves, a scoop of mango, cucumber, and spinach.

MAKES 4 to 6 servings

SUPERFRUIT RECIPE SNAPSHOT: MANGO (WITH SALMON HIGH IN PROTEIN, OMEGA-3 FATS AND CAROTENOIDS; NUTRIENT- AND PHYTOCHEMICAL-ENRICHED SPINACH)
High Nutrient Content: protein, prebiotic fiber, antioxidant A-C-E vitamins, B vitamins, dietary minerals, omega fats
High Phytochemical Content: carotenoids (alpha- and beta-carotene, beta-cryptoxanthin, lutein, violaxanthin); polyphenols (quercetin, gallic acid, gallotannins, rhamnetin, cyanidin and xanthone glycosides, including mangiferin, mainly in mango skin)
Color Code: orange-yellow

Wrapped Roasted Halibut with Superfruits

4 tablespoons canola oil
4 large spinach leaves
2 6-ounce skinless Pacific halibut fillets
6 black mission figs, diced
⅓ cup mandarins
1 sweet onion, diced
About 2 dozen goji berries (wolfberries)
4 cherry tomatoes, halved
2 lemon sections

Preheat oven to 400°F. Line a baking sheet with aluminum foil. Pour 1 tablespoon of the canola oil into the center of each half of the baking sheet. Lay two spinach leaves side by side over each oil drop. Place one fillet on each pair of spinach leaves, and then wrap the spinach around the fish. In a small bowl, combine the remaining 2 tablespoons canola oil with figs, oranges, diced onion, and goji berries. Sprinkle each halibut roll with half of the bowl mixture and tomatoes. Bake about 10 minutes, until halibut flakes. Transfer to dinner plates, and serve with lemon sections.

MAKES 2 servings

 SUPERFRUIT RECIPE SNAPSHOT: FIGS, ORANGES, GOJI BERRIES (WOLFBERRIES) (WITH HALIBUT HIGH IN PROTEIN; NUTRIENT- AND PHYTOCHEMICAL-ENRICHED SPINACH)
High Nutrient Content: protein, prebiotic fiber, antioxidant A-C-E vitamins, B vitamins, dietary minerals, phytosterols, omega fats
High Phytochemical Content: carotenoids (beta-cryptoxanthin, beta-carotene, zeaxanthin, lycopene); polyphenols (anthocyanins, hesperidin, ellagic acid)
Color Code: red-tan, orange

Guava-Kiwi Scallops

6 medium red guavas, halved, seeded, and scooped so there is a cavity
¾ teaspoon ground cinnamon
¾ teaspoon ground cloves
¾ teaspoon sea salt
1 pound fresh or frozen cleaned scallops, cut into bite-size pieces
2 tablespoons canola oil
3 tablespoons lemon juice
2 kiwifruits, sliced (skin optional for extra dietary fiber)
2 lemons, sectioned

Line a baking sheet with aluminum foil. Arrange guava halves on baking sheet. Combine cinnamon, cloves, and salt, and sprinkle mixture over guava. Combine scallops in a bowl with canola oil and lemon juice. Place about 2 tablespoons of scallop mixture into cavity of each guava half. Broil about 8 minutes; remove from broiler, place kiwi onto guava halves, and return to broiler for 2 to 4 more minutes, until kiwi browns. Place two guava halves on each plate, and serve with lemon sections and your choice of vegetables and/or rice.

MAKES 6 servings

SUPERFRUIT RECIPE SNAPSHOT: RED GUAVAS, KIWIFRUITS
High Nutrient Content: protein, prebiotic fiber, antioxidant A-C-E vitamins, B vitamins, dietary minerals, omega fats
High Phytochemical Content: carotenoids (beta-cryptoxanthin, beta-carotene, lycopene); polyphenols (anthocyanins, mixed flavonoids); chlorophyll
Color Code: red-tan, green

Desserts

Dessert time always brings an opportunity for getting an extra serving or two to meet your Color Code and five-a-day requirements. The top twenty superfruits give you a cornucopia of choices for color, flavor, nutrient and phytochemical content, exotic origin, sweetness, and—most of all—fun, to finish your meal on a high note. Share these treats with your dinner partners!

Baked Mango-Banana

1 large firm banana, peeled and halved lengthwise
½ cup mango chunks (peel optional; include for additional dietary fiber)
2 tablespoons canola or olive oil
2 tablespoons dark rum
2 tablespoons grated orange or lemon peel
2 tablespoons brown sugar
½ cup low-fat or nonfat frozen vanilla yogurt

Preheat oven to 350°F. Place banana halves cut-side down in a baking dish. Top with mango. Combine oil and rum, and pour over fruit. Sprinkle orange peel and brown sugar on top. Bake about 20 minutes until brown sugar caramelizes and is crisp. Place ¼ cup yogurt in each of two bowls, and divide mango-banana mixture between bowls. Serve hot.

MAKES 2 servings

SUPERFRUIT RECIPE SNAPSHOT: MANGO
High Nutrient Content: B vitamins, dietary minerals
High Phytochemical Content: carotenoids (alpha- and beta-carotene, beta-cryptoxanthin, lutein, violaxanthin); polyphenols (quercetin, gallic acid, gallotannins, rhamnetin, cyanidin and xanthone glycosides, including mangiferin, mainly in mango peel)
Color Code: orange-yellow

Superfruit Flambé

6 scoops low-fat frozen yogurt
¼ cup triple-fruit (orange-grapefruit-lemon) marmalade
3 packets Splenda, or ¼ cup pineapple juice with diced chunks
½ tablespoon lemon juice
¼ cup water
¼ cup orange, lemon, and/or grapefruit peel, thinly cut or shredded
⅔ cup mixture of mango and papaya chunks
3 tablespoons brandy

Scoop frozen yogurt into three balls for each of two serving dishes, and place in freezer. In a saucepan, heat marmalade, Splenda, lemon juice, and ¼ cup water on medium-high, stirring until syrupy, about 5 minutes. Add fruit peel, mango, and papaya, stirring for 30 seconds. Remove yogurt dishes from freezer. Pour brandy onto fruit mix, and ignite immediately (use caution). Spoon fruit and sauce onto frozen yogurt, and serve.

MAKES 2 servings

SUPERFRUIT RECIPE SNAPSHOT: MANGO, PAPAYA

High Nutrient Content: prebiotic fiber, antioxidant A-C-E vitamins, B vitamins, dietary minerals

High Phytochemical Content: carotenoids (alpha- and beta-carotene, beta-cryptoxanthin, lutein, violaxanthin, lycopene); polyphenols (quercetin, gallic acid, gallotannins, rhamnetin, cyanidin and xanthone glycosides, including mangiferin, mainly in mango peel)

Color Code: orange-yellow

Baked Superfruit Cinnamon Apples

4 medium unpeeled Red Delicious apples or other variety, halved and cored

½ cup mixture of dried blackcurrants, dried cranberries, and raisins

2 tablespoons ground cinnamon

2 tablespoons brown sugar

1 cup low-fat or nonfat vanilla yogurt

Preheat oven to 350°F. Arrange apple halves core-side up in a baking dish, and fill cored-out centers with berry mix. Combine cinnamon and brown sugar, and sprinkle evenly over apples. Pour water into the baking dish to a depth of about ¼ inch. Bake 30 to 40 minutes, until apples are tender when pierced with a fork. Spoon ¼ cup yogurt into each of four bowls, and top with two apple halves. Serve warm.

MAKES 4 servings

SUPERFRUIT RECIPE SNAPSHOT: BLACKCURRANTS, CRANBERRIES, RAISINS

High Nutrient Content: prebiotic fiber, dietary minerals

High Phytochemical Content: polyphenols (anthocyanins—particularly delphinidin and cyanidin glycosides and rutinosides, quercetin, hydroxycinnamic acid, proanthocyanidins, resveratrol)

Color Code: black, red-tan, blue

Guava-Peach Walnut Crisps

1 medium red (strawberry) guava, halved, cored, and seeded

1 unpeeled peach, halved and cored

2 tablespoons chopped walnuts plus 4 walnut halves for garnish

2 tablespoons brown sugar

2 tablespoons grated orange peel

¾ teaspoon ground allspice

½ cup low-fat or nonfat regular or frozen vanilla yogurt

Preheat oven to 350°F. Arrange guava and peach halves core-side up in a baking dish. Combine the chopped walnuts, brown sugar, orange peel, and allspice in a bowl, and sprinkle over fruit. Bake until hot, about 20 minutes. Place one each of the guava and peach halves in two bowls. Scoop 2 tablespoons yogurt onto each fruit half, and top each with a walnut half. Serve warm.

MAKES 2 servings

SUPERFRUIT RECIPE SNAPSHOT: RED GUAVA
High Nutrient Content: prebiotic fiber, dietary minerals
High Phytochemical Content: carotenoids (beta-cryptoxanthin, beta-carotene, lycopene); polyphenols (anthocyanins)
Color Code: red-tan

Frosty Mango-Pumpkin Custard

1 cup low-fat frozen vanilla yogurt

½ cup mango chunks, pureed until smooth

½ can (about 1 cup) pumpkin pie mix

1 tablespoon ground nutmeg

6 walnut halves

Soften yogurt by leaving at room temperature for 10 to 15 minutes or microwaving on high for 20 seconds. Line a six-cup muffin tin with paper baking cups. In a mixing bowl, combine softened yogurt, mango, pumpkin pie mix, and nutmeg. Scoop custard mix into muffin cups, and top each with a walnut half. Cover with plastic wrap and place in freezer for at least 1 hour before serving.

MAKES 6 servings

SUPERFRUIT RECIPE SNAPSHOT: MANGO
High Nutrient Content: prebiotic fiber, antioxidant A-C-E vitamins, B vitamins, dietary minerals
High Phytochemical Content: carotenoids (alpha- and beta-carotene, beta-cryptoxanthin, lutein, violaxanthin); polyphenols (quercetin, gallic acid, gallotannins, rhamnetin, cyanidin and xanthone glycosides, including mangiferin, mainly in mango peel)
Color Code: orange-yellow

Superfruit Hot Tropical Melba

1 8-ounce can peach halves, drained (reserve syrup)
1 can pear halves, drained (reserve syrup)
1 cup mango chunks (peel optional; include for additional dietary fiber)
1 cup papaya chunks, peeled and seeded
1 cup strawberry guava chunks, seeded
½ cup 100 percent orange juice
4 tablespoons frozen orange juice concentrate
½ cup shredded coconut
12 pitted dates

In a large nonstick skillet, combine peaches, pears, mango, papaya, and guava; add the syrup from the peach and pear cans and the orange juice. Stir lightly, and cook over medium-high heat until liquid is reduced by half and thickened (about 10 minutes). Add orange juice concentrate, and continue cooking until concentrate is dissolved. Spoon out fruit into serving dishes, and then add syrup from the pan. Garnish each serving with coconut and two dates. Can be served as a hot topping on vanilla yogurt, light cake, or ice cream.

MAKES 6 servings

Hot Figs

¼ cup 100 percent orange juice with pulp
1 cup low-fat or nonfat vanilla yogurt
16 dried black mission figs
8 mandarin orange segments
3 tablespoons confectioners' sugar

Mix orange juice with yogurt. Spoon ¼ cup of the yogurt mixture into each of four small dessert dishes. Place figs in a microwavable container with 2 tablespoons water (to increase moisture content in the figs), and microwave on high for about 45 seconds (varies according to size of figs and bowl) to make figs hot. Spoon four figs onto each yogurt serving, top with two orange segments, and sprinkle with confectioners' sugar. Serve while figs are still warm.

MAKES 4 servings

High Nutrient Content: prebiotic fiber, antioxidant A-C-E vitamins, dietary minerals

High Phytochemical Content: carotenoids (beta-carotene, beta-cryptoxanthin); polyphenols (anthocyanins, hesperidin)

Color Code: black, orange

Baked Dried Plum Whip

2 tablespoons canola oil

2 cups pitted dried black plums (prunes)

3 packets Splenda

2 tablespoons orange juice

2 tablespoons grated orange peel

½ tablespoon ground cinnamon

2 tablespoons granulated sugar

4 egg whites

2 cups low-fat or nonfat vanilla yogurt

⅓ cup crushed walnuts

⅓ cup goji berries (wolfberries)

⅓ cup red grapes or raisins

Preheat oven to 350°F. Coat a 1½-quart casserole dish lightly with canola oil. In a blender, puree prunes, Splenda, orange juice, orange peel, and cinnamon. Combine sugar and egg whites in a large bowl, and whisk until firm; add prune puree and mix thoroughly. Pile mixture lightly into casserole dish, and bake about 30 minutes, until top is golden brown. Divide yogurt evenly among six serving bowls. Scoop equal portions of baked prune whip into bowls. Combine walnuts, goji berries, and grapes, and sprinkle mixture over each bowl. Serve warm.

MAKES 6 servings

SUPERFRUIT RECIPE SNAPSHOT: DRIED PLUMS, GOJI BERRIES (WOLFBERRIES), RED GRAPES

High Nutrient Content: prebiotic fiber, dietary minerals

High Phytochemical Content: carotenoids (zeaxanthin, beta-cryptoxanthin, beta-carotene, lycopene); polyphenols (anthocyanins, catechins, proanthocyanidins, chlorogenic acid, ellagic acid, resveratrol)

Color Code: red-tan, blue-purple

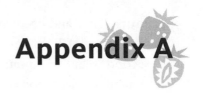

Appendix A

Scientific Foundation Behind Superfruit Antioxidants

THERE ARE THREE CRITICAL foundations to consider in regard to the scientific background of superfruits. To understand why superfruits are exceptional in comparison with more common fruits, here's what you need to know:

- ▶ The antioxidant message
- ▶ Oxygen radical absorbance capacity (ORAC)
- ▶ FDA guidance on antioxidant claims for food or supplement product labels

The Antioxidant Message

You might be asking, "What about the signature we associate most with superfruits—the polyphenol antioxidants?" Let's dispel the antioxidant message about polyphenols right away, with two points.

First, *nutrients* are food components *proved* by science to have health value for humans. Without specific essential nutrients from the diet, people get sick. For example, three antioxidant nutrients established with plentiful science and deemed essential to human health are vitamins A, C, and E—the "ACE" vitamins.

Second, plant compounds called *phytochemicals* are *nonnutrient* components of plant foods that *may* impart health benefits, similar to the pigment antioxidant polyphenols, on the basis of which nearly all superfruit juices are promoted with eye-catching advertisements. Because these phytochemicals await final scientific proof of what they really do in the human body, they are regarded neither as nutrients nor as essential to health.

Both marketers of manufactured superfruit products and the public media have exaggerated the potential antioxidant importance of fruit compounds such as polyphenol pigments (anthocyanins, flavonoids, tannins, catechins, xanthones, and many others). These compounds have antioxidant activity in controlled laboratory conditions, but there is no scientifically confirmed evidence that they have antioxidant roles in the human body.

Interesting new science is giving glimpses that these polyphenols have nonantioxidant roles in which they act in small quantities like hormones or immune modulators to fine-tune genes, enzymes, and receptors involved in cell-to-cell communication. This fine-tuning may be like an "on-off" switch for how diseases start and is likely the reason why eating more fruits and vegetables is often linked to lowering the likelihood of diseases. In other words, insufficient intake of polyphenols from colorful plant foods may leave the switch for starting a disease in the "on" position.

Superfruits and Oxygen Radical Absorbance Capacity

In 2004, food scientists with the U.S. Department of Agriculture (USDA) published a list of antioxidant capacity for one hundred common foods consumed in the United States. This test was branded as ORAC, the oxygen radical absorbance capacity, determined by measuring in a test tube the ability of a food to neutralize free radicals—highly reactive, unstable molecules that, although natural and actually serving useful roles in normal biochemistry, can be damaging if produced chronically in unregulated, high concentrations. Early in 2005, the health food and juice industry picked up on the marketing potential of ORAC for superfruit products by proposing the following premises:

- ▶ Higher ORAC means a more powerful product having greater health benefit.
- ▶ More ORAC in a product should cost more.
- ▶ Juices containing fruits reported with high ORAC in the USDA tables would have the same ORAC value as the actual fruit.

Be wary of such supposed benefits of ORAC; none of these statements is supported by science. Remember that other than for the ACE vitamins, a physiological response or benefit of supposed antioxidant compounds such as polyphenols from fruits or juice has *not* been adequately shown by expert-validated science.

Here are a few facts: (1) ORAC is an artificial benchmark applying only to conditions in a test tube; (2) the ORAC test is fraught with technical inconsistencies as a measurement from lab to lab and often *within* a lab; and (3) there is no concrete, scientific evidence that ingesting more ORAC-enriched foods or superfruit juices means better antioxidant protection in the body or provides any specific health benefit. See Part I for more explanation.

There is good evidence that our bodies react to antioxidant compounds such as polyphenols as "foreign" and unwanted in high quantities, so the body actively metabolizes and excretes them, leaving behind only small amounts—about 3 percent—of the total amount ingested. Also, the concentration of polyphenols remaining in the body hours after a meal is tens to hundreds of times lower than the amount first tested in the lab to determine ORAC, making the lab measurement irrelevant in the human body.

Remember: the way to get the most dietary antioxidants (ACE vitamins) is to eat color-rich fresh fruits, vegetables, and other whole foods regularly rather than only using superfruit juices or extracts that claim to have miraculous health benefits.

Significant Scientific Agreement Built from Accomplishment Within the Research Pyramid

Significant scientific agreement (SSA) is the FDA term that lays out requirements for manufacturers seeking a health claim for a product. It's a comprehensive process that entails all those years of research within the health claims research pyramid (Part I) and qualifies only the most developed new health products for clinical trials, which, if successful, allow eventual health statements on consumer products.

All products not meeting SSA are destined to live in their markets with no credible message about why anyone would want to buy them, in most cases leading to consumer misconceptions about the product. This fact again calls to light the highly successful marketing methods used by manufacturers of superfruit juices that have produced financial rewards in the absence of science proving any health value of these products.

Considering Superfruit Science

The FDA's purpose in requiring SSA is to guard the general consumer from misinformation and to assure *science-based truths* in the marketing of food products. SSA applies to the development of sound science underlying superfruits as health foods with specific actions to improve general health. Qualifying a superfruit product for the health claims research pyramid is based on the following series of questions related to research and product development:

► Have studies appropriately specified and measured the substance that is the subject of the claim?
► Have studies appropriately specified and measured the disease that is the subject of the claim?
► Are any and all conclusions about the substance-disease relationship based on all of the publicly available scientific evidence?
► Does the evidence show consistency across different studies and among different researchers and permit the key determination of whether a change in the dietary intake of the substance will result in a change in a disease end point?

I hope that the information in this appendix has helped you to see that science-based truths about fruits should guide your purchase decisions, a common theme of this book. The hype created especially about superfruit juices having high ORAC and antioxidant benefit is false unless such products contain good to excellent levels of vitamins A, C, and/or E—the only validated dietary antioxidants. With the balance of other nutrients, these vitamins identify true superfruit qualties in packaged or bottled fruit products. On packaged goods, remember to read the Nutrition Facts panel to assure that you are buying a nutrient-rich product.

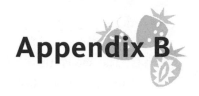

Appendix B

Superfruits
with Edible Seeds

A S THE EMPHASIS OF this book is on the nutrient value of the foods you eat, I want to highlight superfruits with edible seeds so you will be aware of them and will give seed chewing a try. Seeds are Mother Nature's perfect gift-wrapped nutrient package: all the instructions and sustenance needed for the next generation of the plant you are eating are contained in its seeds. Let's accept these seed gifts for their high nutrient value and for the fun of chewing them!

Have a look at this list and see if any of these fruits are already among your favorites—and give the nutrient-rich seeds a try:

- ▶ Blackcurrant
- ▶ Fig
- ▶ Goji
- ▶ Kiwifruit
- ▶ Pomegranate
- ▶ Red grape
- ▶ *Rubus* berries (raspberry, black-berry, boysenberry)
- ▶ Strawberry
- ▶ *Vaccinium* berries (cranberry, blueberry, bilberry)

The seeds in kiwis, figs, and strawberries are barely noticeable and fortunately are plentiful. They are loaded with protein, fiber, valuable omega fats, and micronutrients, so chew as many as you detect while enjoying these fruits.

Among the top twenty superfruits, seeds vary widely in size, number, texture, taste, and "chewability." Those listed here have good crunch quality. The seeds must be chewed to yield the nutrient payload and, for the most part, are tasteless. Some superfruit seeds, such as those in grapes, have a slightly bitter taste, which derives from the polyphenols (proanthocyanidins, tannins, and other phenolic acids) characteristic of the fruit.

Also, open your mind to other fruit seeds that I have enjoyed over many years for their crunch and nutrients—especially protein, essential minerals, omega fatty acids, and fiber: apple, grapefruit, orange, watermelon, and pear. I eat all their seeds and even some of the edible pith and peel, each a great source of dietary fiber!

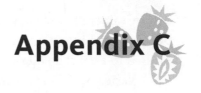

Appendix C

Ten Superfruit Candidates for the Future

S INCE THE MEDIA BUZZ on superfruits began, some forty to fifty fruits have been called "super" by the media, food industry analysts, or manufacturers and marketers of fruit products. Everyone, it seems, wants on the bandwagon of popularity for the word *superfruit*, which stimulates curiosity, rapid translation into sales, and long-term devotion among consumers. Whereas the top twenty superfruits discussed in Part II are established in mainstream global markets, at least ten other fruits are beginning to attract attention and research interest due to their nutrient richness or phytochemical content—these are potential superfruit candidates for the future.

Most of the fruits discussed in the sections that follow are not in the consumer mainstream but are promising for possible development in future superfruit products.

Baobab (*Adansonia digitata*) MAINLAND AFRICA, MADAGASCAR

Whole baobab fruit and extracts are beginning to be sold in the European Union. The fruit has significant nutrient content, possibly with as much vitamin C as oranges, as well as good amounts of calcium and other dietary minerals. The nutrient-rich seeds are used in soups and may also be fermented into a powder condiment, eaten whole after roasting, or pressed to extract an oil rich in omega fats—oleic and linoleic acids.

A variety of folk medicine applications using all parts of the baobab tree indicate that eventually there likely will be extracts tested in disease models by Western scientists.

Bayberry (yangmei, "yumberry," *Myrica rubra*), SOUTHEAST ASIA

Already popularized as a retail juice in the United States and Canada under the name "yumberry," the red bayberry fruit grows on trees as a drupe, meaning it has an outer shell with a single stone seed in the middle; the seed is surrounded by juicy pulp prized for its flavor and color. The rind, pulp, and juice of bayberry are bright crimson.

Analyses of yumberry juice show a cross section of essential nutrients, but levels are not as high as in the top superfruits. More than a hundred reports on bayberry are in the medical research database, most of these identifying polyphenols extracted from the tree bark or leaves. Ellagic acid is the dominant polyphenol in yumberry juice among many isolated polyphenols, including high contents of tannins and anthocyanins.

Anticancer activity was demonstrated in laboratory tests using extracts of leaves from a related species, *Myrica gale,* and a delphinidin (anthocyanin) extract showed anticancer and antiviral activity in test-tube experiments.

Black Chokeberry ("aronia," *Aronia melanocarpa*) CANADIAN PRAIRIES, NORTHERN UNITED STATES (ALSO EASTERN EUROPEAN NATIONS)

The chokeberry (better known in recent years as aronia) is probably the most anthocyanin-enriched and therefore most astringent and bitter-tasting fruit native to North America. Aronia juice is already in commercial use to add flavor and dark purple color in blends with grape, blueberry, and cranberry juices. Aronia mostly grows wild and is systematically farmed on a sizable scale in eastern Europe. Owing to its bitterness, aronia is not widely sold as fresh produce.

Given its exceptional polyphenol content, aronia holds continuing basic research interest for a variety of disease models, nearly all of which are in early-stage research. Two human studies from Poland indicate potential use for aronia extracts in treating hypertension in patients with metabolic syndrome, as well as in reducing symptoms or risk of diabetes.

Animal experiments show that aronia lowers blood cholesterol levels in a high-fat diet, reduces blood glucose and triglyceride levels, inhibits blood clotting and onset mechanisms for cancer, and alleviates inner-eye inflammation.

Although these same effects could be demonstrated with other polyphenol-enriched berries, the relatively higher concentrations of anthocyanins and proanthocyanidins in aronia simplify sourcing these polyphenols to one plant.

Black Elderberry (*Sambucus canadensis*, *Sambucus nigra*)
EASTERN CANADA, NORTHERN UNITED STATES, CENTRAL EUROPE

A staple of aboriginal lore, black elderberry is often called "nature's medicine cabinet" in recognition of the numerous phytochemicals found in the fruit's beautiful, fragrant white flower, deep purple berry skin, pulp, seeds, leaves, and tree bark.

Black elderberry fruit has significant nutrient content, qualifying it for candidate superfruit status. Its thick berry skin and seeds contribute a high percentage of dietary fiber and polyphenols, and the fruit is rich in vitamin C, B vitamins, and several dietary minerals. Likely due to its sourness and strong flavor, black elderberry, however, has not become widely popular. Consequently, it is not farmed on a significant commercial scale, and so in most of Canada and Europe, it grows wild in ditches and forest perimeters.

Its research foundation is sound. Over the past sixty years, there have been eight hundred reports on basic laboratory studies involving elderberry. Preliminary evidence reveals that the fruit's diuretic properties are possibly useful for controlling body weight, and there is research showing antiviral, immune-stimulating, anticancer, and cardiovascular effects.

Black Raspberry (*Rubus occidentalis*, *Rubus leucodermis*)
NORTHWESTERN UNITED STATES

Due to the denser content of polyphenols, particularly deep purple anthocyanins, giving them an almost black color and sourness when ripe, black raspberries are less popular than their more common red raspberry cousins. Most varieties have a strong astringent (sour) flavor so are unlikely to become a favorite as fresh produce.

In the past decade, medical research programs at Ohio State University have focused on black raspberries as potential therapeutic agents against several forms of cancer, especially those of the mouth and throat. A slowly dissolving lozenge or some other orally available format containing a black raspberry preparation has promise to allow prolonged contact with tissues needing therapeutic treatment, such as for leukoplakia, a precancerous lesion common in smokers.

The dense anthocyanin and fiber contents of this berry species are the most likely therapeutic benefits. Related studies are just entering human clinical trials, but the foundation of basic research and probable physiological mechanisms of action are promising for further development of consumer products or drugs.

Despite such optimism, overall consumer demand is low, and this species of raspberry has not been systematically cultivated sufficiently to be resistant to common plant fungi. Consequently, black raspberries are not farmed extensively and their total cultivated acreage in the United States remains low.

Cape Gooseberry (*Physalis peruviana*) PERU, COLOMBIA
(ALSO SOUTH AFRICA AND AUSTRALIA/NEW ZEALAND)

This relatively large, golden berry is bigger than a grape but smaller than a cherry tomato; has a sweet, pleasant taste with little sourness; and probably is low in organic acid content. Increasingly seen in fresh produce markets, the Cape gooseberry seems to have a growing consumer demand as a novelty, as it should for its attractive uses in fresh fruit cocktails, salads, chutneys, pies, jams, and puddings.

As a relative of the tomato, potato, and goji plant family, *Solanaceae*, the fruit is notable for its high carotenoid (provitamin A) content, evident by its attractive yellow-orange pigmentation. It appears to get its name either from where it was first cultivated on the Cape of Good Hope, Africa, or from the interesting physical "cape" wrapping each berry, a paperlike mantle that overlies and protects the ripening fruit like a loose jacket.

Research to date indicates that forty chemical compounds make up the Cape gooseberry's flavor profile, and it has a good range of micronutrients, fatty acids, and carotenoids. Anti-inflammatory activity has been demonstrated in laboratory experiments on tumors, as has inhibition of experimental inflammation of the eye, similar in efficacy to a topical steroid.

Durian (*Durio kutejensis*) THAILAND

One of those fascinating creations of nature, durian is called the "king of fruits" by Thais. It stimulates the senses for its somewhat offputting fragrance contrasted against delicious, complex taste.

Durians are mostly eaten fresh or are simply boiled with sugar or cooked in coconut water and served with rice or mixed vegetables or as a relish. Durian pulp may be canned in syrup, dried and packaged, or made into a canned paste for export. Seeds may be eaten after cooking with sugar as a confection or fried with coconut and spices as a side dish. Leaves and roots may be eaten in salads.

Durian nutrients are diverse at good levels, two exceptions being omega fats and vitamin E, which are highly enriched in the fruit and seeds. Polyphenols include quercetin and caffeic, p-coumaric, and hydroxycinnamic acids. A topic in the medical literature since the 1960s, durian displays no specific tested or published antidisease properties.

Indian Gooseberry (amalaka, amla, *Phyllanthus emblica*)
INDIA

Used for centuries in Asian traditional practices, Indian gooseberry is a sour, bitter fruit that is often steeped in salt water and turmeric to make a tart tea. The fruit is reputed to have exceptional vitamin C content. One report shows that there is 0.45 gram of vitamin C per 100 grams of pulp (about 75 times more than an orange), but this measurement may be obscured by high tannin density. The fruit contains several other polyphenols as well.

Indian gooseberry is the subject of ongoing basic research, demonstrating inhibitory effects against bacteria and experimental viruses and modification of gene expression in osteoclasts (bone cells) possibly associated with arthritis and osteoporosis. Other preparations of leaves, tree bark, or fruit show actions against laboratory models of inflammation, cancer, and diabetes. A human pilot study in Taiwan demonstrated that the extracts from this fruit reduced blood levels of an oxidative stress marker, prostaglandin, in patients with failing kidneys.

Muscadine Grape (black or bronze scuppernong, *Vitis rotundifolia*) SOUTHEASTERN UNITED STATES

If more acres of this fascinating grape species existed, there would likely be a fresh rebirth of the dark grape juice and wine industries. Having a thick, deep purple skin influencing its entire phytochemical profile, the muscadine is a research dream for its richness of dietary fiber, tannins, ellagic acid, anthocyanins, and resveratrol (apparently, however, some muscadine cultivars, possibly the gold varietal, are mysteriously low in resveratrol content). One of the first grape species cultivated in North America, muscadines have remained geographically restricted to the southeastern states from Texas to Florida and north to the Carolinas.

Muscadines are distinguished by their sourness and toughness for chewing, accounting for the reputation these grapes have as being suitable mainly for wine or for artisan jams, juice, and flavors in alcoholic beverages. The seeds especially are concentrated with proanthocyanidins and resveratrol, which may facilitate development of further grape nutraceutical products.

Laboratory studies have shown positive effects from muscadine polyphenols against test-tube or animal models of inflammation and of blood, colon, and prostate cancers. A 2009 study at the Mount Sinai School of Medicine in New York demonstrated that muscadine wine was more effective than cabernet in reducing neuropathology in a mouse model of Alzheimer's disease.

Saskatoon (*Amelanchier alnifolia* Nutt) CANADIAN PRAIRIES

If you asked western Canadians for their favorite berry in pies, jams, syrups, and yogurt, the saskatoon would likely be their answer. It's the only berry after which a city has been named—Saskatoon, Saskatchewan, largest city in the province. Increasing exports of dried and sugar-infused saskatoons to Britain have extended the popularity of this berry.

Saskatoon berries have a nutrient profile similar to that of the highbush blueberry, containing good levels of dietary fiber and the essential minerals calcium, iron, and manganese. Particularly noticeable when eating these berries, saskatoon seeds are rich in micronutrient value, including omega-3 and -6 oils and vitamin E. As the berry pulp and skin content of phytochemicals is high in anthocyanins, proanthocyanidins, tannins, and catechins, research progress has been mainly on inhibiting mechanisms of inflammation.

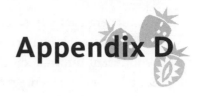

Appendix D

Bibliography, References, and Author's Other Publications

Online News Sources for Superfruits

FoodNavigator: foodnavigator-usa.com
Food Processing: foodprocessing.com
Functional Ingredients: functionalingredientsmag.com/fimag
Natural Products Information Center: npicenter.com
Natural Products Insider: naturalproductsinsider.com
Nutraceuticals World: nutraceuticalsworld.com

Consumer Guidance and Nutrition Facts

Centers for Disease Control and Prevention, "Fruits and Veggies—
More Matters": fruitsandveggiesmatter.gov
Gourmet Sleuth, kitchen volume and metric conversions: gourmet
sleuth.com/conversions.htm
Harvard School of Public Health, "Food Pyramids: What Should You
Really Eat?": hsph.harvard.edu/nutritionsource/what-should-you-
eat/pyramid-full-story

Micronutrient Fact Sheets, Feinberg School of Medicine, Northwestern University: feinberg.northwestern.edu/nutrition/fact-sheets.html

Micronutrient Information Center, Linus Pauling Institute, Oregon State University: lpi.oregonstate.edu/infocenter

Nutrient Data Laboratory, Agriculture Research Service, U.S. Department of Agriculture, "Oxygen Radical Absorbance Capacity (ORAC) of Selected Foods—2007": ars.usda.gov/SP2UserFiles/Place/12354500/Data/ORAC/ORAC07.pdf

Nutritiondata.com, an excellent resource for nutrients of many foods: nutritiondata.com

2009 Change4Life Program, British Department of Health: nhs.uk/change4life/pages/make.aspx

U.S. Department of Agriculture, National Nutrient Database: ars.usda.gov/services/docs.htm?docid=8964

World's Healthiest Foods, in-depth nutrient profiles and excellent supporting essays for plant foods and their components: whfoods.com

World's Healthiest Foods, "How Healthy Nutrition Builds Health, Starting with the Cells" (graphics): whfoods.com/genpage.php?tname=faq&dbid=19#faqdiscussion

Color Code

Heber, D. *What Color Is Your Diet?* New York: ReganBooks, 2001.

Joseph, J. A., D. A. Nadeau, and A. Underwood. *The Color Code: A Revolutionary Eating Plan for Optimum Health*. New York: Hyperion, 2002.

General

Blue Zones Community. bluezones.com/about.

Brownell, K. D., and K. B. Horgen. *Food Fight: The Inside Story of the Food Industry, America's Obesity Crisis, and What We Can Do About It*. New York: McGraw-Hill, 2004.

Clinicaltrials.gov. U.S. National Institutes of Health. clinicaltrials.gov.

Ho, L., et al. "Heterogeneity in Red Wine Polyphenolic Contents Differentially Influences Alzheimer's Disease–Type Neuropathology and

Cognitive Deterioration." *J Alzheimers Dis.* 16, no. 1 (January 2009): 59–72.

Joffe, M., and A. Robertson. "The Potential Contribution of Increased Vegetable and Fruit Consumption to Health Gain in the European Union." *Public Health Nutr.* 4, no. 4 (August 2001): 893–901.

Lea, E. J., D. Crawford, and A. Worsley. "Consumers' Readiness to Eat a Plant-Based Diet." *Eur J Clin Nutr.* 60, no. 3 (March 2006): 342–51.

Li, T. S. C., and T. H. J. Beveridge. *Sea Buckthorn: A New Medicinal and Nutritional Botanical.* Ottawa: Agriculture and Agri-Food Canada, Publication 10320E, 2007.

Liu, L., Y. Wang, K. S. Lam, and A. Xu. "Moderate Wine Consumption in the Prevention of Metabolic Syndrome and Its Related Medical Complications." *Endocr Metab Immune Disord Drug Targets* 8, no. 2 (June 2008): 89–98.

McCullough, M. L., and W. C. Willett. "Evaluating Adherence to Recommended Diets in Adults: The Alternate Healthy Eating Index." *Public Health Nutr.* 9, no. 1A (February 2006): 152–7.

Murphy, S. P. "Using DRIs as the Basis for Dietary Guidelines." *Asia Pac J Clin Nutr.* 17, Suppl. no. 1 (2008): 52–4.

Popkin, B. M. "Global Nutrition Dynamics: The World Is Shifting Rapidly Toward a Diet Linked with Noncommunicable Diseases." *Am J Clin Nutr.* 84, no. 2 (August 2006): 289–98.

Pratt, S. G., and K. Matthews. *SuperFoods Rx: Fourteen Foods That Will Change Your Life.* New York: HarperCollins, 2004.

Pratt, S. G., and K. Matthews. *SuperFoods HealthStyle: Proven Strategies for Lifelong Health.* New York: HarperCollins, 2006.

Sohn, E. "Superfruits, Super Powers?" *Los Angeles Times*, March 10, 2008.

Swinburn, B. A., I. Caterson, J. C. Seidell, and W. P. James. "Diet, Nutrition, and the Prevention of Excess Weight Gain and Obesity." *Public Health Nutr.* 7, no. 1A (February 2004): 123–46.

Time. "The Fat of the Land—Ancel Keys." January 13, 1961. time.com/time/magazine/article/0,9171,828721-1,00.html.

UNICEF—United Nations International Children's Emergency Fund, Nutrition. unicef.org/nutrition/index_bigpicture.html.

van't Veer, P., M. C. Jansen, M. Klerk, and F. J. Kok. "Fruits and Vegetables in the Prevention of Cancer and Cardiovascular Disease." *Public Health Nutr.* 3, no. 1 (March 2000): 103–7.

WebMD. webmd.com.

Wikipedia. wikipedia.org.

World Health Organization. "Joint Health and Nutrition Strategy to 2015." who.int/nmh/media/speeches/nmh_adg_speech_unicef_eb.pdf.

World Health Organization. "The World Health Report." who.int/whr/2002/chapter5/en/index5.html.

Willett, W. C. *Eat, Drink, and Be Healthy.* New York: Simon & Schuster, 2001.

Health Claim Approvals and Health Research

AREDS, the Age-Related Eye Disease Study. U.S. National Eye Institute, National Institutes of Health. nei.nih.gov/amd.

European Food Safety Authority. efsa.europa.eu.

U.S. Food and Drug Administration. "A Food Labeling Guide," FDA-qualified health claims about foods, appendix C. cfsan.fda.gov/~dms/2lg-xc.html.

U.S. Food and Drug Administration. Food Labeling, Nutrient Content Claims, Definition for "High Potency" and Definition for "Antioxidant" for Use in Nutrient Content Claims for Dietary Supplements and Conventional Foods. cfsan.fda.gov/~dms/hpotguid.html.

Mediterranean and "Portfolio" Diets

Alexandratos, N. "The Mediterranean Diet in a World Context." *Public Health Nutr.* 9, no. 1A (February 2006): 111–7.

Barberger-Gateau, P., C. Raffaitin, L. Letenneur, C. Berr, C. Tzourio, J. F. Dartigues, and A. Alpérovitch. "Dietary Patterns and Risk of Dementia: The Three-City Cohort Study." *Neurology* 69, no. 20 (November 13, 2007): 1921–30.

Belahsen, R., and M. Rguibi. "Population Health and Mediterranean Diet in Southern Mediterranean Countries." *Public Health Nutr.* 9, no. 8A (December 2006): 1130–5.

Jenkins, D. J., et al. "Long-Term Effects of a Plant-Based Dietary Portfolio of Cholesterol-Lowering Foods on Blood Pressure." *Eur J Clin Nutr.* 62, no. 6 (June 2008): 781–8.

Jenkins, D. J., C. W. Kendall, A. Marchie, A. L. Jenkins, P. W. Connelly, P. J. Jones, and V. Vuksan. "The Garden of Eden—Plant-Based Diets, the Genetic Drive to Conserve Cholesterol and Its Implications for Heart Disease in the Twenty-First Century." *Comp Biochem Physiol A Mol Integr Physiol.* 136, no. 1 (September 2003): 141–51.

Naska, A., et al. "Fruit and Vegetable Availability Among Ten European Countries: How Does It Compare with the 'Five-a-Day' Recommendation? DAFNE I and II Projects of the European Commission." *Br J Nutr.* 84, no. 4 (October 2000): 549–56.

Regmi, A., N. Ballenger, and J. Putnam. "Globalization and Income Growth Promote the Mediterranean Diet." *Public Health Nutr.* 7, no. 7 (October 2004): 977–83.

Trichopoulou, A. "Traditional Mediterranean Diet and Longevity in the Elderly: A Review." *Public Health Nutr.* 7, no. 7 (October 2004): 943–7.

Trichopoulou, A., and E. Critselis. "Mediterranean Diet and Longevity." *Eur J Cancer Prev.* 13, no. 5 (October 2004): 453–6.

Trichopoulou, A., A. Naska, and E. Vasilopoulou. "Guidelines for the Intake of Vegetables and Fruit: The Mediterranean Approach." *Int J Vitam Nutr Res.* 71, no. 3 (May 2001): 149–53.

Willett, W. C. "The Mediterranean Diet: Science and Practice." *Public Health Nutr.* 9, no. 1A (February 2006): 105–10.

Willett, W. C., F. Sacks, A. Trichopoulou, G. Drescher, A. Ferro-Luzzi, E. Helsing, and D. Trichopoulos. "Mediterranean Diet Pyramid: A Cultural Model for Healthy Eating." *Am J Clin Nutr.* 61, Suppl. no. 6 (June 1995): 1402S–1406S.

Mediterranean Recipes and Lifestyle

Cloutier, M., and E. Adamson. *The Mediterranean Diet*. New York: Harper, 2001.

Woodward, S. *The Classic Mediterranean Cookbook*. Montreal: Reader's Digest Press, 1995.

Author's Superfruit Publications and Presentations

Peer-reviewed citations on Medline, U.S. National Library of Medicine, search = gross pm. pubmed.gov.

The Berry Doctor's Journal, free consumer-education newsletter on superfruit research and nutrition. berrydoctor.com

Gross, P. M., X. Zhang, and R. Zhang. *Wolfberry: Nature's Bounty of Nutrition and Health*. Charleston, S.C.: Booksurge Publishing, 2006.

"Nature's Colorful Gifts." *Vista* 46, May–June (2006), 20.

"Wolfberry: Nutritious Superfood." Natural Products Insider, August 21, 2006. naturalproductsinsider.com/articles/681feat05.html.

"Exploring Exotic Antioxidant Superfruits." Natural Products Insider, October 16, 2006. naturalproductsinsider.com/articles/472/6ah169431 758327.html.

Article series on berries and superfruits. Natural Products Information Center. npicenter.com/news/drpaulgross_articles.aspx.

E-zine article series on berries and nutrition. http://ezinearticles .com/?expert=dr._paul_gross.

"Superfruits Take Center Stage: Defining An Emergent Category", Natural Products Information Center, February 26, 2007. npicenter .com/anm/templates/newsATemp.aspx?articleid=17826&zoneid=201.

"Tracking Market Meteors: Exotic Superfruits." Natural Products Insider, November 16, 2007. naturalproductsinsider.com/articles/ tracking-market.html.

"Exotic Superfruits: Literature Update." Natural Products Insider, November 16, 2007. naturalproductsinsider.com/articles/ 7bh16125940.html.

"Deciphering Superfruits and Their Future Market Impact." SupplySide East, Secaucus, N.J., April 28, 2008. Speaker.

"Berry Research Breakthroughs: Ten Trendsetters of 2007–8." Natural Products Information Center, June 2, 2008. npicenter.com/anm/templates/newseditorial.aspx?articleid=21343&zoneid=43.

"Superfruits Have Signatures." Natural Products Information Center, August 6, 2008. npicenter.com/anm/templates/newsatemp.aspx?articleid=21604&zoneid=251.

"Noni: Superfruit or Health Myth?" Natural Products Information Center, November 10, 2008. npicenter.com/anm/templates/newsatemp.aspx?articleid=22601&zoneid=251.

"Superfruit Validation: Clinical Trial Status Confirms Scientific Strength." Virgo Publishing Webinar Series, December 2008. Speaker. naturalproductsinsider.com/webinars/superfruits_webinar.html.

Superfruit Validation and Product Strategies." Nutracon and ExpoWest, New Hope Natural Media, March 2009. Organizer, chair.

"FDA's Antioxidant Guidance: Is This the End of the Road for Marketing Polyphenols as Antioxidants?" Nutraceuticals World, March 2009. nutraceuticalsworld.com/articles/2009/03/new-roles-for-polyphenols.

"Qualifying Criteria for Superfruit Status." SupplySide East, Secaucus, NJ, April 27, 2009. Speaker.

"The Mangosteen Controversy." Natural Products Information Center, May 21, 2009. http://www.npicenter.com/anm/templates/newsATemp.aspx?articleid=24082&zoneid=273.

"Comprehensive Criteria for Superfruit Status (Determining How 'Super' Those Fruits Really Are)." Natural Products Insider, July 20, 2009, 46–50. naturalproductsinsider.com/articles/comprehensive-criteria-for-superfruit-status.html

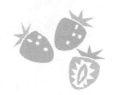

Index